The
HEALING
POWER
of
COLOR

The
HEALING
POWER
of
COLOR

How to Use Color to Improve
Your Mental, Physical, and
Spiritual Well-being

BETTY WOOD

Destiny Books
Rochester, Vermont

Destiny Books
One Park Street
Rochester, Vermont 05767

LIBRARY OF CONGRESS CATALOGING-IN-PUBLICATION DATA
Wood, Betty, 1929-
    [Healing power of colour]
    The healing power of color : how to use color to improve your mental, phys-
ical, and spiritual well-being / Betty Wood.
        p. cm.
    Originally published: The healing power of colour.
Wellingborough: Aquarian, 1984.
    Includes index.
    ISBN 0-89281-400-4
    1. Color—Psychological aspects. 2. Color—Therapeutic use. I. Title.
BF789.C7C66 1992
133—dc20   92-3632
                                                                        CIP
Printed and bound in the United States by Capital City Press

10 9 8 7 6 5

Destiny Books is a division of Inner Traditions International

CONTENTS

INTRODUCTION

In a book about color and color healing, it is important to understand that we do not have to visually perceive color for it to have some effect on us. Color on its own and in the form of light continuously affects those more subtle senses and autonomous processes that ultimately play such a significant part in our lives.

Color-blind people, for instance, may be totally unable to see colors such as red and green and, at worst, may only see a gray world. The totally blind from birth may only have the haziest idea of what we mean by color. However, Professor Harold Wohlfarth, a photobiologist at the University of Alberta and president of the German Academy of Color Science, believes that color has a physiological effect. In an experiment he found that light had an "identical" influence on the blood pressure and pulse of two blind children as it had on seven sighted children. He contends that light colors can cause reactions in one or more of the brain's neurotransmitters. But it also seems that in certain cases it can affect other parts of the body, if recent experiments in China and Russia are anything to go by. It is claimed in these instances that a number of people have been able to see colors and read with different parts of their bodies other than their eyes.

Each of us sees color in a slightly different way, although we might call it by the same name. Even so, two people may disagree as to whether a color is, say, blue or lilac. Some cultures have no words for complex colors and find the primary colors the most attractive.

"Let there be light" is the primal cry of many creation myths, for without the action of the "Sun God" life would never have manifested as it did. As we know, of course, light has a very important effect on all growing things and on all living creatures, including humans, on whose reproductive processes it has a significant effect. In the stronger form of sunlight, it promotes the formation of vitamins in the body, especially vitamin C, and in some instances causes vitamin deficiency—as can happen after overexposure to certain types of fluorescent lighting. Light striking the retina appears to influence the pineal gland's synthesis of melatonin, a hormone that helps determine the body's output of serotonin, a neurotransmitter.

According to Alexander Schauss, director of the American Institute for Biosocial Research the electromagnetic energy of color affects the pituitary and pineal glands and the hypothalamus, all of which have a profound influence on the bodily system. While it is still a matter of controversy among scientists and psychologists, they all have to agree that the sections of the electromagnetic spectrum we cannot see, such as X-rays, microwaves, and ultraviolet rays, definitely affect the physical body, so it does not seem impossible that the section of the spectrum that we can actually see can also affect us in various ways.

Life would be somewhat flavorless without the stimulation of color— how we use it can tell us a lot about ourselves and may tell other people even more. If we are unwise in our color schemes we may give quite the wrong impression to others, or we may be so drab as to slip by unnoticed and wonder why we never make an impact! Color, therefore, affects the whole of our lives—in our homes, our places of work and play, our dress and our behavior. Later in this book we shall perhaps gain insight as to why we choose certain colors in preference to others and how, by careful use of color, we can change the mood of a room or even the attitude of another person toward us.

Psychologists disagree between themselves about the significance of color in the human personality but, as in the Lüscher Test (which will be discussed later) there seems to be a correlation between color and personality. Much of this may be due to cultural influences and upbringing, but if we go back to prehistoric days, we can see how important color was to early humans and how it has evolved. Human intuition is a very useful guide also, and in the long term will probably prove more reliable than a dozen psychological personality tests.

Color has texture, taste, and feel—some people even hear it as a corresponding musical note: slow, heavy music conjures up blues and darker colors while rapid tempo is at the red end of the spectrum; high-pitched tones bring light colors to mind and low-pitched tones bring dark colors. Psychologists think this is probably based on inherited traits but have no satisfactory explanation. To some people, every day of the week is a different color, which never changes throughout their lives; numbers are different colors; and names evoke different colors—for example, all Michaels are green and all Elizabeths, blue.

We also carry around with us our own personal electrical field known as *aura*. This is somewhat similar to the earth's aurora, with positive north at the head and negative south at the feet. The most brilliant display is usually around the head, which can be seen to some degree by most people after a little practice and knowing what to look for. The aura is an important indicator of health and mood and state of mind; it can be rapidly assessed by someone particularly gifted in this way. For us lesser mortals, however, if we can only partially see or even not see the aura at all, there is no cause for dismay—unless particularly unaware, most of us can sense an aura and react automatically as an attractive or hostile auric field approaches us.

In short, we are subtly, and sometimes dramatically, influenced by color all the time. A bright orange or red poster comes forward to grab us, while the gentler colors of blue and green appear to draw back and lead us on. Advertisers catch the eye by careful arrangement of shapes and colors, much as the flower attracts a bee.

Finally, how we see and use color in all its varied shades, tones, and hues may be but a reflection of our inner memories. Some of the most beautiful examples of color—an opalescent dawn of gold and rose, the luminous blue of an evening sky, sunlight through stained glass windows, or a rainbow spanning the heavens—may well bring to our minds a far away remembrance of some other realm, where light and color weave patterns at which we can only guess. Our dreams and meditations bring back a glimpse of these, and, used wisely in our quest for healing and wholeness, they can only have a beneficial and harmonizing effect.

1
COLOR
IN OUR PAST

If we search through time in an endeavor to trace the evolution of color awareness and sensitivity, to a great extent we can only speculate. Such speculation is, however, often validated by discoveries in archaeology and anthropology. Our earliest known ancestors, Cro-Magnon man and Neanderthal man, have only left small traces of their existence—stone tools, bone implements, fragments of human skeleton, and occasional burial places. The most exciting finds have been the cave paintings, executed with superb craftsmanship and colored with natural materials—various pigments to which prehistoric humans had fairly easy access.

Of these early attempts at coloring, the most obvious conclusion is that humans looked around themselves at the environment and the creatures and the plants that flourished in abundance; at the sky, the sun and the moon, the rivers and the sea; and at themselves. They saw the colors of the earth, of fire and blood and water, fur and feathers in all their great variety, and brightly-hued reptiles and insects. They found materials at hand such as red ochre, an oxidized earth that ranges in color from yellow to purple, also known as bloodstone or hematite. Neanderthal skeletal remains have been found lying in a bed of red ochre; sometimes the bones were painted with ochre, a practice still carried on today, for instance, by Australian Aborigines.

This pigment was not regarded simply as a means of decoration but as very special material symbolic of various sacred powers and principles needing to be invoked for aid and protection. In Africa stone tools dating back to prehistoric times have been found adjacent to old mine workings dating back some 50,000 years. Archaeologists have been reluctant to admit that these mines were worked by prehistoric humans, because they were not known to have discovered the use of metal ore. Instead the overlooked fact is that they may have been mining for pigment instead. Now, in a recent book by Lyall Watson called *Lightning Bird* (see Further Reading), there appears a most convincing argument that early humans did, in fact, mine for pigment in much the same way as do present-day Africans.

Lightning Bird is the true story of a young man, Adrian Boshier, who early in life determined to go to Africa and explore it on foot. He became a legend in his time not only for his snake-handling abilities but also for his knowledge and experience of native culture. A priestess-diviner, Rrasebe, took him under her wing and taught him many of her secrets. One day she took him to some caves and told him how she remembered her father working with his paints. He would grind some white stone, charcoal, and red earth and mix them with water and other liquids. Having obtained the desired result, he would then paint traditional designs and patterns on the rocks. "Throughout Africa," says Lyall Watson, "color plays an important role in symbolism, particularly that related to medicine." As a result of this knowledge and the actual discovery of prehistoric tools in Swaziland, Adrian Boshier interested a well-known paleontologist, Professor Dart, who gave him advice and help. It seems likely from their joint research, and comparison with tools Professor Dart had found in Zambia, that shamanistic priests and diviners still use similar tools and methods of extraction for pigments such as crystals of manganese dioxide and pyrolusite (also very much valued in ancient Egypt) as their forefathers did thousands of years before.

In Africa, important colors are black, red, and white. Not too surprisingly, black is the color of night, death, excrement, and illness, while white is daylight, life, food, and good health. Red indicates transformation—the red of sunrise is a move toward health; the red of sunset, a decline into disease. However, for the Masai, black is a very important color with many positive aspects. It symbolizes the color of thunderclouds, for example—a much desired sight in the dry season.

What applies to peoples in Africa could also well apply to similar cultures in other parts of the world—Europe, Asia, and the Americas. One of the first colors most likely to have made a great impact on humans was red—the color of blood and fire. Blood was the source of mysterious power, the life force, irreplaceable and mystical, the mainstream of life. A blood sacrifice was the greatest thing humans could give to their gods—their blood or, preferably, something or someone's very life energy. We who consider ourselves civilized can hardly imagine now the effect of such a ceremony upon a group of people whose lives and beliefs were so very basic, although to some extent the blood sacrifice still goes on in some parts of the world. We may even have our modern equivalent in the daily slaughter on the roads. Fire and its association with the sun, its warmth and protection so essential, its destructive power and mystery, made it one of the most potent sacred symbols.

Black, with its negative associations, also was a very special color, signifying all those fearful, dark, and hidden forces of nature and the unknown from which early humans had to protect themselves. Its opposite, white, represented the lighter, happier, positive qualities that made life enjoyable.

It does not take too much imagination to connect yellow with the sun and thus symbolize another form of life. Gradually, no doubt, more colors became available from minerals, seeds, plants, and insects. Lapis lazuli, turquoise, and various gemstones possibly gave painters ideas for coloration so that by the time of the earliest civilizations there was a wide range of materials available for painting and personal decoration.

Color was absolutely essential for its protective and magical qualities—it drove off evil spirits and encouraged good ones to help and protect. The shamans or priests of the tribe were probably responsible for rock and cave paintings, and they made the choice of colors and pigments that set the scene for everyone else. Shamanism, the oldest known religion on earth and most likely the precursor of all later cults, is derived from humans' deepest roots and oldest, most basic beliefs and feelings. Early humans and most people living close to nature were, and still are, highly sensitive to their natural environment, and in their dreams and visions they perceived the "gods" and the various colors associated with them. There has been some talk of various rock paintings in Africa depicting spacemen, but it seems much more realistic to consider that these strange figures, with "globes" around their heads and various ritualistic implements in their hands, are denizens of the dream world and part of a remarkably consistent pattern experienced by native seers around the world, the archetypes of humankind's inner life and of the great life principles at work in the universe.

Dr. R. M. Bucke, author of *Cosmic Consciousness,* a classic well worth reading on many counts, has put forward an interesting theory regarding the evolution of color sense in humankind. He takes the analogy of childhood development and compares this to the gradual evolution of early humans. In the child, he maintains, memory appears a few days after birth, then after a few weeks, simple consciousness and curiosity develop; at a few years, use of tools and finally self-consciousness, followed shortly by awareness of color and fragrance. No doubt this varies with individual children and may likewise vary with individual cultures.

Dr. Bucke quotes an early researcher, Lazarus Geiger (1880), who pointed out that it could be proved by examination of language that as late in the life of the race as the ancient Aryans, perhaps not more than 15,000 or 20,000 years ago, humans were only conscious of, and only perceived, one color. That is to say, they did not distinguish be-tween blue sky and green trees and grass, or brown or gray earth. All these colors might be described by the one word "black." Adolphe Pictet (1877), another researcher, reported that he found no names of colors in primitive Indo-European speech. Max Mueller (1887), a language researcher, found no Sanskrit root whose meaning has any reference to color. At a later period, when the main part of the *Rig Veda* (early Sanskrit writings) was composed, red, yellow, and black were recognized as three separate colors; still later white was added to the list, and eventually green, but throughout the *Rig Veda,* the *Zend Avesta,* the Homeric poems with their "wine-dark" sea,[1] and the Bible, claims Dr. Bucke, the color of the sky is not once mentioned. He therefore concludes that blue was not recognized. Although this is an intriguing idea, it is not altogether convincing, especially from the point of view of blue not being recognized. For instance, in the Bible blue is mentioned many times—Ezekiel 23:6 mentions horsemen "clothed with blue, captains and rulers" and "blue and purple from the Isles of Elishah." Apart from Joseph's coat of many colors, in Exodus 25:4 offerings are described as "blue, and purple, and scarlet . . . and gold." In Esther 1:6 "white, green, and blue hangings" and royal apparel of "blue and white" are described. Ezekiel likens God unto a rainbow: "As the appearance of the bow that is in the cloud in the day of rain, so was the appearance of the brightness round about." And on another occasion God was seen standing on "As it were a paved work of sapphire stone, and as it were the very heaven for clearness." So it seems rather unlikely that in biblical days people were unable to see or describe the color blue. Green also appears many times in the Bible—"green pastures" in Psalm 23:2, "green herbs" in Genesis, while Jacob (Genesis 30:37) "took him rods of green poplar." Many other colors also have extensive mention.

Basically, however, we come back to red, black, white, and yellow as the earliest colors. When Dr. Leonard Woolley excavated the ziggurat at Ur, one of the oldest buildings in the world, he found that it was built in four stages, with the lowest black and the uppermost red. Pursuing his theory, Dr. Bucke states that the English word "blue" and the German word "blau" are said to descend from a word that meant black, and the Chinese hi-u-an, which now means sky blue, formerly meant black. Nil, which in Persian and Arabic means blue, is derived from the name Nile, which meant Black River and of which the Latin Niger is a form. Dr. Bucke believed that under the designation "red" were included white, yellow, and all intermediate tints; while under "black" were included all shades of blue and green.

There is a rapid decrease in the energy of light waves as we pass along the spectrum from red to violet. If, as Dr. Bucke suggests, the eye evolved according to the power of a light wave to excite vision, it would seem natural that red, with energy rays several thousand times as great as blue and violet, would be the first color perceived, followed by yellow, then green, and so on to violet. He cites various studies undertaken by researchers to determine the incidence of color blindness. It seems that 4 percent of European males (and 0.25 percent of females) suffer from it to some extent; the incidence is slightly lower for Chinese males at 3 percent. However, among the Japanese the incidence is much lower and it might be surmised, rightly or wrongly, that as a culture their color sense evolved at a very early date.

Dr. Bucke considered color-blindness to be a modern phenomenon of possible atavistic origin and not properly belonging to this age. It is an intriguing thought that perhaps in the far distant future humankind will acquire an extended color range, maybe even comparable to that of the bee.

Once the great civilizations began to develop, color, with its important magical qualities, was extensively used. One likes to think also that maybe by then, if not before, homo sapiens had also developed a sense of beauty and did not regard color simply as a practical necessity. As far as orthodox archaeology tells us, the Mesopotamians (Chaldeans) are perhaps the earliest recorded civilizations, as such, living in cities and organizing themselves to quite a degree of sophistication. The Chaldeans were believed to be the ancient Magi—masters of magic and astrology who dedicated their temples to planetary gods of the heavens. James Fergusson, in his *History of Architecture in All Countries* (1893), tells us that they decorated these temples in the appropriate colors depending on which god had his abode there. Herodotus refers to what seems to be the great temple of Nebuchadnezzar at Barsippa, which was 272 feet square at its base.

It rose in seven stages, each one set back from a central point. It was found that this temple was dedicated to the seven planets and was decorated with the colors of each. Thus the lower stage was black, the color of Saturn; the next, orange for Jupiter; the third, red for Mars; the fourth, yellow for the sun; and the fifth and sixth, green and blue, respectively, for Venus and Mercury; the upper stage was probably white for the Moon, whose place in the Chaldean system was extremely important. Present-day astrologers disagree somewhat as to planetary colors, as will be discussed later.

Next came the Egyptians. Their temples, tombs, and presumably their homes were decorated inside and out with bright, clear colors of black, red, yellow, green, blue, and purple. "Color" meant the same as substance,[2] of which color was an important part. If one said of the gods that one could not know their color, it meant that one could not know their substance, their essence. Emotional qualities were attributed to certain colors—red was aggressive and suggested danger, but it was also life-giving. It would be placed alongside blue,which was subdued and yet flowing out to infinity.

The gods and goddesses had their special colors denoting their various qualities. Osiris, for instance, was sometimes referred to as "the great green" and was often painted green because of his associations with fertility, resurrection, and death. He was also known as "the Black One," no doubt due to his association with the underworld. Black, as in earlier cultures, was a reference to death and the netherworld but also of rebirth and ressurection. Bread made from white grain and beer from red were food and drink in the netherworld. In other instances the two colors became opposites, as in the case of hippopotami where the red male animal and the white female were regarded as hostile and helpful, respectively. The Egyptians not only decorated their buildings and sculptures but also themselves, for example, using red paint and jewelry for a particular festival, probably much the same as present-day Hindus scatter various colored substances, particularly red and yellow, at religious festivals. While Egyptian art remained stylized for the most part over the several thousand years of their culture, there were periods when the country was in a state of instability and art suffered accordingly. They have nevertheless bequeathed to us a legacy that still influences our color utilization today—most notably, perhaps, in our choice of religious ceremonial clothes, which are often scarlet. Red often symbolized life and victory, and red and white together (as in the St. George's flag) expressed wholeness and perfection. The White Crown of Upper Egypt and the Red Crown of Lower Egypt were worn together to symbolize the unity and balance of the whole country.

Sometimes red took on a more negative aspect, as it was also the color of Set, god of the desert and of the typhoon, the negative force in Egyptian mythology. Set was thought to have red eyes and red hair (the color of the desert) and thus a person "with a red heart" was considered to be in a rage; "to redden" meant the same as "to die." There was a red lake of fire in the underworld in which the damned were punished—another legacy for us! "To do red things" meant to do evil, while "to do green things" meant the opposite.

White became expressive of earthly omnipotence, a way of symbolizing sacred things, and was the color of purity and sanctity. It was also the color of joy, and a cheerful person was referred to as "white." Gold symbolized the sun and all its various attributes and was the natural choice of color for the god Ra. The god Amun was colored blue because of his cosmic associations.

Early Egyptians and Greek temple decorations may have appeared rather garish to our eyes, accustomed as we are to the mellow gold-beige of the present-day ruins. But many examples of Egyptian decoration are still around for all to see, and it takes no great stretch of imagination to apply this to the Greek and Roman temples of later date. As with the Egyptians, Greek marble statues were often highly colored, with red lips, and eyes decorated in yellow, green, and blue, often with eyelashes as well. Particularly impressive are those statues with eyes made of precious stones, which must have been most awe-inspiring when first seen gleaming out of the darkness of a tomb, shining like the eyes of a cat. Some find it rather painful to consider that the exterior of the Parthenon, for instance, was similarly embellished with bright colors of red, blue, yellow, gold, and black decorating the cornices, friezes, and columns. The Romans, as usual, followed suit, and their gods determined color choices. Purple, or a magenta color, was reserved for the emperor in his role as the personification of Jupiter. Although unfortunate for the inhabitants, it is our gain that Pompeii and Herculaneum were sufficiently preserved under volcanic ash for us to see the wonderful paintings and artwork of that time. Likewise, in the palace of Minos in Crete, dating back to 1600 B.C. and before, many restorations can be seen of the original wall paintings and decorations in red, yellow, blue, brown, and black, with red and black the predominant colors.

Another ancient people to whom color was significant were the Chinese. In fact, their various dynasties were represented by colors—brown for the sun, green for Ming, yellow for Ch'ing. Predictably enough, the emperor wore blue when worshiping sky deities and yellow when worshiping earth deities. The Chinese had five primary colors—red, yellow, black, white, and green, which in turn corresponded to the five elements (fire, metal, wood, earth, and water), the five happinesses, the five virtues, the five vices, and the five precepts of faith. Their subsequent discovery of jade in all its varied and delicate shades no doubt enlarged their color sense immensely. Today we seem to think we are the only people with regard for the beauty of nature and the value of wild creatures, but one has only to look at the accurate and expressive drawings of animals, birds, and all other creatures as portrayed by the artists of these early cultures to see that, although portraying all of nature with a true and unsentimental eye, they drew and painted, one might say, from the heart.

Red, as in almost every other culture, was regarded in China as the positive, masculine essence, and yellow as the earthly and feminine principle. Buildings were often painted red, symbolic of the south, sun, and happiness, with yellow roofs symbolic of the earth. When a home was built, red firecrackers were exploded and a piece of red cloth was suspended to promote happiness and well-being. Green pine branches were placed on top of the scaffolding to deceive wandering evil spirits into thinking they were passing over a forest. Red and yellow are the marriage hues for the Orient in general, Egypt,

Russia, and the Balkans. It is not surprising that red in China is regarded as the luckiest of colors, representing the sun and the phoenix bird. Orange also represents love and happiness, while blue denoted the Azure Dragon of the East, the heavens, clouds, and the spring. While it would be tedious to enumerate colors as used by every culture since these early days, it might be useful to see the correspondences between various widespread areas of the world. Red is almost universally regarded as the most positive, creative, and life-giving color. It does, however, have its negative side, as we have seen. In Celtic mythology red meant disaster and is symbolic of martyrdom, cruelty, and zeal in the Christian church.

Black is associated with primordial darkness and everything negative. It also signifies time and is associated with the dark aspect of the Great Mother (especially as the Hindu goddess Kali, who is Kala) and with time. Black or blue-black is the color of chaos, of storm clouds. In Christian tradition it symbolizes the Prince of Darkness, hell, death, and so forth, as well as spiritual darkness and the unconscious. In Hebraic Cabalistic tradition it symbolizes mercy and understanding, but the general consensus of opinion seems to incline to the idea of black as a negative, frightening color.

White, naturally enough, usually represents the opposite. While it has associations with both life and death, it usually stands for wholeness, purity, and innocence and is a most sacred color. Used by the Chinese, and sometimes the Romans, for mourning, it nevertheless has associations with spiritual authority. Buddhists regard it as the color of self-mastery, while the ancient Egyptians, who wore a lot of it, considered white and green to be symbolic of joy. White and silver also relate to the moon and the unconscious, feminine side of humankind.

Nearly everywhere yellow stands for the sun, along with gold, and signifies divine power, enlightenment, and immortality. In Hinduism gold is life, truth, light, immortality, the seed, and the sign of Agni (the Hindu god of fire). The Buddhists regard it as the color or renunciation, desirelessness, and humility and often wear ochre robes, which were believed to have been adopted because they were originally worn by condemned criminals and outcasts. Yellow is a color of mostly happy associations—of sun and brightness, light and life. But, like other colors, it has its negative side, and dark yellow can signify treachery, faithlessness, and betrayal.

Next, comes blue and all its associations of sky and water. Most cultures connect blue with truth, revelation, wisdom, loyalty, fertility, constancy, and chastity. Blue is the color of the great deeps, the feminine principle, the Great Mother. In the West the blue cloak of the Mother Goddess is a vastly protective and comforting symbol, evocative of peace, compassion, and healing. We even incorporate a little bit of it in our "something borrowed, something blue" for the bride. Blue is a color that one can sink into, a view with which most ancients might agree. It is the color of infinity and infinite peace, the wisdom of Dharma-Dhatu in Buddhist thought. Blue denoted the bard or poet in Celtic mythology, the raincloak of Indra, the war and fertility god of the Hindus. For Cabalists it is the color of mercy. Everyone seems to love blue, although at times it can denote coolness and remoteness.

Along comes green, with its associations of nature in all its aspects, the cycle of birth and death. In Buddhist ideology vernal green denotes everything pertaining to life, while pale green signifies death. In Christian thought also, vernal green denotes immortality, hope and growth of the Holy Spirit in humans, triumph over death, and the annual ressurection of spring after winter, while similarly pale green signifies Satan, evil, and death. The most noteworthy quality of green is possibly that of transformation, life and death, abundance on one hand and unripeness, immaturity, and even decay on the other. It has soothing and harmonizing qualities and neutralizes the pushiness and energy of red. In Cabalism green stands for victory; it is also the sacred color of Islam. Strangely enough, in the West it is often regarded as unlucky because of its links with "the Little People." It is their color, and it might upset them to see humans wearing it. Or perhaps the Christian church frowned on its associations with fertility, being only too aware of the call of Pan, which can lure your soul away, never to be redeemed!

Brown, and earthly color and one of the oldest, is usually symbolic of the Earth and, although frequently used in paintings, does not seem to have been particularly sacred. Like black, brown can denote death to the world and negation of personality, as when used by some religious orders. It also can symbolize penitence and a renunciation of earthly things.

Violet and purple probably came a little later on the scene, and the discovery of the Murex shellfish no doubt gave a wonderful boost to the Phoenician economy. From this shellfish they acquired the dye for their "Tyrrhenian purple" so much in demand for royalty and for ceremonial robes. For the Aztec and Inca cultures purple stands for majesty and sovereignty, while in the West it is the color of Jupiter and religious devotion. It usually seems connected with spiritual values and was reserved for certain privileged people. Today, still used for special occasions, it is a rather "heavy" color to wear and needs a strong personality or grand occasion to carry it off successfully. Lesser shades of violet and lilac often have spiritual connotations.

The colors discussed in this chapter were the main colors used by early cultures, but, of course, orange, gray, pink, and all their variations were also used. Gold and silver were inevitably the sun and the moon, the one rich and warm and the other cool and delicate. In Cabalism gray represents wisdom, orange represents splendor. Many ancient peoples gave specific colors to the four corners of the earth, but these vary from place to place between such widely diverse cultures as Old Irish, Mayan, and North American Indians. As used in Navaho sand paintings today, white represents the universal cosmic energy; black, the great void from which all comes; red, life and energy; yellow, the sun; and blue, spirituality.

From these early days, color awareness took off with a splendor which has rarely been matched since. The Byzantines revelled in the lavish use of color with a richness and brilliance that may cause some to prefer the simplicity of earlier times. And then came the Renaissance, its painting and sculpture lighting up the whole of the Middle Ages as if after a period of spiritual darkness all the candles in the world had been lit. Many secrets of color have been lost as master painters, glassblowers, and stained glass artists guarded their recipes so carefully that no one was able to repeat them. A barrister named Charles Winston

(1847) managed to rediscover some of the medieval constituents of colored glass.[3] He and Dr. Medlock of the Royal College of Chemistry found, for example, that the most beautiful blue was obtained not from lapis lazuli, as had been previously thought, but from cobalt. Kazakh (U.S.S.R.) scientists have likewise recently rediscovered the formula for the glazing used to decorate medieval architectural monuments after studying the multicolored patterns of the fourteenth-century artist, Ahmad Yasavi. They established that the old mural painters used sand and clay as basic materials, with other necessary components obtained from the ashes of "sarychob" roots.

Stained glass in England owes much of its wonderful brilliance to the various recipes used by generations of craftsman, but it also owes a great deal to the climate with its grayer light, which shows stained glass to much greater advantage than does the brilliant sunshine of the Mediterranean and the Far East. Colored glass was regarded as particularly precious from early monastic days. Theophilus, a German monk writing in the first half of the twelfth century, in his treatise *On Divers Arts* considerable detail about the making of windows, but carefully leaves out chapters that give precise instructions for the coloring of glass with copper, lead, and salt. This was one of the secret recipes so jealously guarded. June Osborne, author of *Stained Glass in England,* writes that "In religious terms, light was a symbol of vital importance, used to describe the quality of spirit itself." And stained glass, while much more expensive than plain, "could be used to fill the congregation with a sense of mystery and vision and also had the function of glorifying God for his own sake." "Like and intelligent enquirer, " wrote Theophilis, "I have labored to inform myself, by all methods, what invention of art and vitality of color may beautify a structure and not repel the light of day and the rays of the sun." Specimens of colored glass have been found in Saxon monastic buildings of the seventh or eighth century, and there is a remarkable range of color, considering the possibility of a rather limited range of materials available. Several shades shades of red, turquoise, viridian, eau-denil, four different shades of yellow, violet and a very pale violet, and white glass streaked with purple, are among the colors used. Francis

Wilson Oliphant (1855), a glasspainter among other things, said "the power of glass... to convey color is quite unique; no kind of painting can at all come up to it. Glass is . . . a luminous material, full of points which catch the light like the facets of a diamond."

Many of the great painters have also striven after this quality of luminosity, particularly for religious paintings, and again there have been many secret recipes, some of which have been lost and some rediscovered. Glass luster artifacts also reflect this quality, and it is obviously something integral in the human being that requires this reminder of realities other than the ordinary, everyday appearance of things, as mentioned in the Introduction. In the *Phaedo,* Socrates describes the "real earth" and says of it that "the colors which we know are only limited samples, like the paints which artists use; but there the whole earth is made up of such colors, and others far brighter and purer still . . . even these very hollows in the earth, full of water and air, assume a kind of color as they gleam amid the different hues around them, so that there appears to be one continuous surface of varied colors." Gems also have this peculiar quality of luminescence, a hidden fire in their depths, which again stirs some long-forgotten memory. Ancient literature is full of such remarks as ". . . has the appearance of a sapphire" or ". . . was the color of amber," or again ". . . a rainbow round the throne, in sight like unto an emerald" (Revelations). The description of the New Jerusalem includes walls of jasper, garnished with all manner of precious stones, and, of course, we all know of the pearly gates!

Josephus, the Jewish historian in the first century A.D., associated white with earth, red with fire, purple with water, and yellow with air. However, 15 centuries later Leonardo da Vinci stated his color preferences as "white for the representative of light, without which no color can be seen; yellow for the earth; green for water; blue for air; red for fire; and black for total darkness." Some of these colors are still included in astrological tradition, as with yellow for Mercury and air and things intellectual; red for Mars and fire and energy.

So fashions and preferences tend to change and evolve—in one era nobles, warriors, the middle class, and peasants tended to wear distinguishing colors, as in early Aryan cultures. At other times certain colors have been reserved for specific trades and professions, as today in law, religion, and the armed forces. Faculties at universities and colleges have their special colors, children at school have their team colors, and colors are extremely important in many sports, not only in order for contestants to identify one another, but for the audience also to identify them. All over the world colors of symbolic significance have been woven into tapestries and beadwork; painted on icons, walls, pottery, and stonework; and incorporated into inlay work, stained glass, glass vessels, and jewelry, not only for ornamentation and visual enjoyment, but for the practice of sympathetic and protective magic in all its aspects, and ultimately and simply for the glory of God.

To return to the Chaldeans for a moment, their traditions have no doubt influenced later generations up to the present, particularly those engaged in magic and astrology. Cabalism is one example where the use of color is essential to "set the scene" for magical working. Other esoteric traditions in the West also use colors for their rituals and workings, as can be seen from the teachings of such organizations as The Order of the Golden Dawn, which has given rise to many similar and breakaway movements. For example, if one wishes to conjure up the power of the sun god in his guise as Appollo, or Ra or whatever, gold and yellow would be the prominent colors to use—altar cloths, flowers, ritual implements, clothing, ornaments, and so on would all repeat the theme of gold and yellow. Likewise with the moon, where silver, white, and perhaps touches of green or violet would be essential. All the planetary gods have their special colors, although these vary a little between different esoteric and astrological traditions. Mostly, however, colors tend to be grouped as follows:

Sun—gold, bright yellow. Leo, its astrological sign, is assigned red, gold, and sometimes yellow-green.

Moon—silver, white, and emerald green and often green and gray in smokey hues for its astrological subject Cancer.

Mars—red, of course, crimson, scarlet, and similar shades. Aries, its zodiacal subject, often has red and white as its colors. The old barber-surgeon's pole (a Martian occupation if there ever was one) is striped red and white, which may therefore not just be an allusion to blood and bandages. Mars is also the ruler of Scorpio and here the darker shades of red apply.

Venus—blue, blue-green, and turquoise. Venus is the ruler of two astrological signs, Taurus and Libra, and all three share the colors.

Mercury—yellow or orange, while some opinions add lilac and off-white. Mercury is another somewhat volatile ruler of two signs, Gemini and Virgo, who share these colors.

Jupiter—purple, of course, sometimes violet or russet reds. This royal planet shares its colors with its subject Sagittarius.

Saturn—olive green and gray, sometimes dark greens and black. Its astrological subject is the reputedly sober Capricorn.

Uranus—electric blue, pale greens, or citrine, always light colors are favored by this planet and Aquarius, two somewhat erratic areas of the zodiac.

Neptune—dark blue, indigo, grays, green. The mystical planet happiest in Pisces, Neptune has been assigned several colors but all of a filmy nature. Some traditions use pink or coral.

Pluto—yellow, pale green, or navy blue have been suggested. This enigma has not yet been assigned to any particular area and therefore is still a bit undecided; you'll have to use your own feelings as a guide to this one.

Earth—our own planet is often assigned lavender blue or white.

If you want to work your own rituals, not only are there many books giving guidelines and color correspondences in this respect, but you can use your own intuition. After studying the qualities of the "god" or "cosmic principle" you wish to invoke, set up your own color scheme for the working which most appeals to you, both aesthetically and intellectually, and which "feels right." You may find some helpful ideas in later chapters.

2
Color
in Our Present

Outer Color and Science

Objectively speaking, there are two main ways in which we are visually aware of color. We perceive a colored object by the light reflected from it, and we also see colored light that comes through transparent matter, such as stained glass or when a beam of sunlight passes through a prism and white light is split into colors of the rainbow—red, orange, yellow, green, blue, indigo, and violet. Not until 1672 when Sir Isaac Newton described his experiments in passing sunlight through a glass prism was it possible to explain the appearance of the colors of the rainbow. Now we know that visible light is just a very small part of the vast spectrum of radio waves, varying in length and speed, as in the case of visible light—from red, the slowest and longest, to blue, the fastest and shortest.

Before we go into the subject of radio waves, however, it might be as well to take a brief look at the mechanism of seeing color. Without involving too much technical detail, it can be said the human eye interprets light rays (electromagnetic energy) by an interaction of the optic nerves with the brain, involving a system of rods and cones in the retina. The eye then externalizes these rays as colors. It seems that there are about 1,000 distinguishable hues and more than 2,000 tints and shades perceived by the human eye. For the colorblind this is severely limited. Experiments have found that 1 person out of every 55 cannot tell red from green, and 1 person out of 50 confuses brown and green. Pink and yellow look alike to some people, and blue and green are similar for others. A very few people see everything in black and white.

Life holds hazards for the colorblind—many cannot distinguish colored lights at airports, on ships, and at traffic and railway signals, except by guesswork. A friend who was a pilot during World War II said he couldn't understand why ground control "overreacted" sometimes when he came in to land. It turned out that he couldn't distinguish the red warning light from the green go-ahead. At that time he was in his early 20s and had no idea that he was colorblind. The red electrical "live" wire thus holds particular dangers for the colorblind, which is presumably why Common Market regulations have changed it to brown, with blue for neutral and striped green and yellow for earth.

Various colors are produced by light waves of different lengths. Objects do not possess a fixed color of their own but depend on the light reflected from their surfaces for color. Leaves on plants appear green because they reflect green rays and absorb all other light, but if a leaf is held under red light it will appear black. All things are thus any color—yellow, blue, or brown, according to their ability to absorb certain light rays and reflect others. Transparent objects are colored by their ability to screen out certain rays—as in blue glass, for instance, when only blue rays pass through it. A transparent object that transmits all colors equally well, such as pure water in small quantities, is said to be colorless.

Colors differ in hue, which is the difference between blue and red, or green and yellow. Colors of the same hue may differ in value or intensity, owing to the difference in the amount of light they reflect; or in purity, according to the amount of grayness in the colors. Surfaces capable of reflecting all color rays appear red in red light, blue in blue light, and white in daylight. Other surfaces absorb all light rays and reflect none. These are black. Adding white to a standard hue, as in red becoming pink, tints the color, while adding black forms shades. Artists' colors, and all the other dyes, paints, and inks used by humans, produce color because of their ability to reflect different light waves. From just a few substances a great many colors can be created. Blue, red, and yellow are called primary colors because from different combinations of these all other colors may be produced. Colors form complementary pairs such as red and green, yellow and violet, blue and orange. One of the tricks our eyes can play on us is to cause us to see a complementary color image. This is where difficulties can arise in "seeing" the aura (discussed in a later chapter). Someone wearing bright red will often appear to have a green aura around them and so on. If you stare fixedly at a bright green object and then look away quickly at a white surface you will see a replica of the object in red. This is because the eye soon tires of one color, so that when looking at a white surface or pale background, it welcomes the other colors and responds less to the color that has produced fatigue. In fact, if you stare at anything too fixedly the eye becomes tired and one of the most common colors then seen is a greenish-blue—another point to bear in mind if you are looking at auras.

As mentioned, visible light is only a very small part of the electromagnetic spectrum; in fact, it covers only 1/60th of the known radio spectrum (figure 1). Long radio waves are used for radio communications, induction heat, and photography where they can penetrate great distance and heavy atmospheres and take pictures where the human eye can hardly see. Next comes radiant heat, laser beams for cutting, and holography. Long waves can measure several thousand feet from crest to crest, whereas the wave length of, say, sodium (yellow) light is very short—about 45,000 waves to an inch. At the far short end of the spectrum are X-rays, gamma rays, and cosmic rays. Most of these rays pass through our bodies harmlessly, although overexposure to X-rays, gamma rays, microwaves, laser beams, and so forth is extremely dangerous, if not lethal.

Visible light also penetrates deeply into animal and human muscle, even as far as the central organs if the light intensity is strong enough. Scientist E. E. Brunt and his associates caused light to penetrate the

Figure 1: *The Electromagnetic Spectrum*

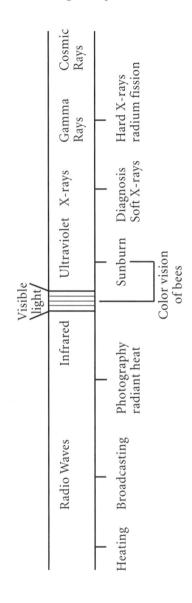

skulls of sheep, dogs, and rabbits and demonstrated "that light does reach the temporal lobes and hypothalamus in a variety of mammalian species"[1]—no doubt in the human being also. Another scientist, W. F. Ganong and his colleagues concluded that "environmental light can penetrate the mammalian skull in sufficient amount to activate photoelectric cells embedded in the brain tissue." "This means," says Faber Birren, "that light is essential to a healthful and normal life and that nature has evolved ways in which it affects the body through the tissues of the skin, the eyes, and even the skull itself."

The human being and all other creatures also emit light and radiation waves of their own, quite apart from those creatures that have a luminous appearance, such as glowworms, fireflies, and deep-sea fish. Dr. Glen Rein, a biologist from St. Bartholomew's Hospital in London, said in a lecture at the College of Psychic Studies in April 1983 that the human body emits many radio waves, including visible light (the latter partly as the aura). Dr. Rein has worked with healers and found that healing energy and electromagnetic energy have a significant effect on enzyme activity and neurotransmission. He described how crystals emit and electric current under pressure and how electromagnetic energy can be fed into them. He pointed out that there were crystals in the pineal gland, for instance, and it could be assumed form this that if electromagnetic energy is fed into them in some way, it could possibly have profound effects on one's health.

It is therefore evident that not only radio waves but visible light has a significant effect on humans and all other creatures. Even the lower animals, such as amoebae, react to light, some preferring weak light or shade or very little light at all. Light has a profound effect on human and animal sexual cycles. For instance, the starlings of Piccadilly who are exposed to all the brilliance of advertisement and street lighting, were found to have active reproduction organs at a time when their country cousins outside the city were sexually impotent. One could, of course, put it down to the influence of Eros but somehow other scientific tests appear to refute this!

Farmers have found that chickens lay more eggs in winter if extra light is provided, and weasels, rabbits, and ferrets have been induced to grow winter fur coloration during the hot days of summer by manipulating the amount of light available to them. In his fascinating book *Light, Color and Environment,* Faber Birren reports that similar results have been achieved with goats, whereby breeding and milk supply can be controlled. Apparently, short days induce breeding and long days inhibit it.

Birren also mentions a case study in which mink were reared behind different colored plastic windows by scientist John Ott.[2] Normally, mink are very aggressive, particularly during the mating period. Ott found that mink kept behind pink windows became increasingly aggressive and vicious and there was less frequency of pregnancy after mating. However, mink kept behind blue plastic became more docile and could be handled easily. All females became pregnant after mating. It also seems that the human male is excited by red radiation and pacified by blue.

Most mammals are, from our point of view at least, visually colorblind, although color vision exists in insects, fish, reptiles, birds, and apes. All, however, react to color whether they can "see" it or not. Rodents kept under blue light were found to have normal growth rates, but under pink or red, appetite, and subsequently weight, increased. Prolonged exposure to pink resulted in death to mice, however, Ott kept 1,000 mice in separate colonies with three different forms of lighting—bluish fluorescent, pinkish fluorescent, and natural daylight. (Natural daylight can, of course, vary greatly in intensity depending on the time of day and season of the year.) He found that under natural light offspring produced were 50% male and 50% female; under blue light offspring were 70% female and 30% male; and under pink the results were 70% male and 30% female! The use of bluish artificial light (presumably in order to breed more females with thicker coats) is commonplace among commercial breeders of chinchilla.

Plants also are significantly affected by light intensity, length of day, and color even more than by temperature and moisture conditions. By the process of photosynthesis, light causes carbon dioxide and water to unite in the presence of chlorophyll to form simple sugars. Most of these are food for the plants as well as for the animals and humans who subsequently eat them.

Birren tells us that Tessier of France[3] (1783) was one of the pioneers in investigating the growth of plants by means of colored light, and he recorded marked growth differences. Then later, General A. J. Pleasanton of Philadelphia upset the horticultural applecart by propounding various startling theories regarding the use of blue (which he regarded as the most important color) glass panes in his greenhouse. He claimed great yields of grapes with this system, although Birren feels these were exaggerated. In 1895, C. Flammarion reported the best effects with red light, and in 1902 L. C. Corbett found that red light had a markedly stimulating effect on lettuce growth. These and various other investigators have been followed by more scientifically oriented experimenters.

It is now standard practice among many gardeners to regulate the amount of light their plants receive. John Ott found that chrysanthemums could be made to flower any month of the year by regulating their exposure to light. He conducted many experiments with colored light and filters. He found that when the male and female flowers of the pumpkin, for instance, were exposed to bluish daylight fluorescent light, the former withered and the latter flourished. Regular fluorescent light caused the female flowers to wither but not the male. Blue light and filters caused morning glory to open, but warm light shrivelled them up. It would seem therefore that by taking careful note of the time of year and prevailing conditions in which a plant flourishes, it should, in theory, be possible to grow almost anything out of its normal season and environment (except that to my mind something grown out of season never has the flavor or texture of naturally grown vegetables and fruit). Even so, the effects of light and color on plants are most intriguing and they are a wonderful example of the interaction of various forces combining to produce the world in which we live.

It appears that, like other organisms, plants are most responsive to red and blue and inactive to yellow and yellow-green. Red causes lettuce seed to sprout, but infrared sends the sprouts to sleep again. Red also inhibits flowering of short-day plants (presumably autumn or winter plants) and assists flowering of long-day plants (late spring and summer plants). If one works for any length of time in an illuminated greenhouse, then weak green illumination is best for both human eyes and for plants, as it does not cause any adverse reaction for either. Stuart Dunn of the University of New Hampshire found that tomato seeds produced interesting results when grown under different colored lamps. Warm white lamps produced the highest yield (this is probably comparable to natural sunlight); next came blue and pink lamps. Green and red lamps produced low yield while experimental high intensity red lamps produced the highest yield of all. Nowadays, special lamps are available to growers wishing to get their plants off to an early start.

Theo Gimbel[4] found that primary red filter light initially overstimulated plant growth, which later became stunted; the plant had an elastic texture and bitter taste. Green started off well but ultimately disintegrated. Those under a blue filter did even better than those under clear light, growing thickly and higher than had been anticipated. He does not, however, name the plants grown, so be cautious if you are thinking of trying out blue filters on any exotic seeds you may have acquired, as they might well require a different type of light altogether.

Another interesting point is revealed by Birren, who points out that "some plant life has an aura!" Apparently, in 1923 Alexander Gurwitsch[5] wrote of discovering what he called "mitogenetic energy," whereby an onion, for example, emits rays in the shorter ultraviolet region of the spectrum. Although of very low intensity, it has tangible and measurable existence. This has been verified by subsequent investigators but is still something of a mystery, with various scientists holding completely opposing opinions.

Faber Birren, who has hundreds of articles and many books published on color and its implications, cites many interesting pieces of research on the effects of light and color on the human organism. He quotes H. L. Logan, a leading lighting engineer, who points out that light dilates blood vessels, increases circulation, and thus rids the body of toxins and lightens the load on the kidneys. Hemoglobin in the blood is increased by light and decreased by darkness. Light also induces hormonal processes through the activation of endocrine glands. Another researcher, Richard J. Wurtman, produced evidence that the stimulation of light may come through the eyes, but effects can also be triggered through the skin and subcutaneous tissues. "It seems clear that light is the most important environmental input, after food, in controlling bodily function," states Wurtman.

Wurtman also found that blind girls tended to menstruate earlier than girls with normal vision, and he thought this was possible because "in the absence of retinal response to light (this) produces an imbalance which results in earlier menstrual function." Among Eskimo women, menstruation may cease during the season of long arctic nights, possibly because lack of light leads to a natural form of human hibernation.

We can thus understand that color and light affect the whole of life. How effective then are the claims for healing by color? In this chapter we shall examine some of the more orthodox claims for color therapy since the days of Neils R. Finsen.

Niels R. Finsen of Denmark was the pioneer of light research. He believed that visible red light would prevent scar formation in cases of smallpox, and in 1896 he wrote of the actinic (chemical action) properties of sunlight and founded a light institute for the cure of tuberculosis. He was awarded a Nobel Prize in 1903 and later reported startling cures among some 2,000 patients, using both sunlight and ultraviolet light.

Birren tells us that Downs and Blunt of England discovered the bactericidal action of ultraviolet radiation in 1877. In India rickets is fairly common, possibly because of the custom followed by women and children in higher castes who stay indoors most of the day. There is also an incidence of rickets when people of sunnier climates move to Britain and are similarly deprived of sunshine and vitamin D. Ultraviolet radiation is essential in these cases—it produces vitamin D, prevents rickets, destroys germs, and effects certain necessary chemical changes in the body. Ultraviolet radiation can be used to cure various skin diseases.

In the United States ultraviolet radiation has become standard treatment for psoriasis. Fish in aquariums can be cured of some virus diseases by radiating them with a certain amount of ultraviolet light. It works equally well for other animals. It can also be used for irradiating food stuffs such as lard, oil, and milk to form vitamin D, but oddly enough cod-liver oil loses its main properties after irradiation. Ultraviolet radiation also tends to increase protein metabolism and helps reduce sugar level in the blood of diabetics. However, short-term overexposure can cause skin damage and a painful eye condition known as photokeratitis. Long-term effects include skin cancers and cataracts of the eyes. Infrared long waves are very hazardous to the human eye and also seem to have a deleterious effect on the action of Vitamin D.

There are many scientists who are convinced that color, as well as light, has a more powerful impact on health and behavior than previously thought. Color is used nowadays in treating a variety of diseases. For instance, within the last 10–15 years, baths of blue light have replaced blood transfusions for about 30,000 premature babies born each year with potentially fatal neonatal jaundice. (U. S. figures). However, blue lights irritate the nurses working in these wards and many hospitals have added gold lamps to impart a soothing quality.[6] In general it has been found that working with babies is greatly helped by blue light, which lessens crying and overactivity.

White fluorescent light, in conjunction with photosensitizing drugs, is widely used to help heal herpes sores. Some unlucky people develop a skin rash if exposed to visible blue or violet light—this may be caused by aftershave lotions, cosmetics, and such or the allergic effect of eating certain foods or by handling allergy-creating substances that interact with light. Nowadays there are effective drugs to counteract unwanted radiation. Certain dyes are also used for such conditions as psoriasis and herpes, which are then exposed to visible light. In this way visible light can help heal damage caused by invisible ultraviolet light. One dye, chrome yellow, has been found to be particularly effective[7] when used in conjunction with a blue-violet light source. The use of porphyrins (sensitizing agents) has had favorable effects on some minor forms of cancer and tumors, whereby they accumulated at the afflicted area and any cancerous tissue is "severely damaged when exposed to visible or near ultraviolet light." The use of dyes and light for skin afflictions is still very controversial and many scientists do not consider them useful.

In Russia, where for considerable time they have been experimenting with and using color therapy, extensive use is made of ultraviolet light, particularly in cases where they suspect miners might be susceptible to black lung disease. They also use it to supplement schoolroom light. As a result it is claimed that children grow faster than usual, with fewer colds and improved work performances.

Some investigators working on the effects of color on bodily activities claim that red light increases muscular activity, blood pressure, respiration, and heart rate. In fact, red appears to be a very disturbing color for anxious people. Blue has the reverse effect, reducing blood pressure and eyeblink frequency, and subsequently any eye irritations, and it is thought to be conducive to sleep. Red might be useful in arousing people troubled with reactive depression or neurasthenia. In some instances red seems to improve growth; it also causes a decrease in blood sugar and has been recommended for some cases of eczema. Gestalt psychologists, such as Heinz Werner, Krakov, Allen, and Schwartz, have found that loud noises, strong odors, and tastes, tend to raise the sensitivity of the eye to green and to decrease sensitivity to red. Birren states "It may thus be generalized that color affects muscular tension, cortical activation (brain waves), heart rate, respiration, and other functions of the autonomic nervous system."

It may affect some people even more dramatically. Birren tells of a woman with a cerebellar disease who had a tendency to fall unexpectedly. When she wore a red dress such symptoms were more pronounced. He points out that tremor and some conditions of Parkinson's Disease "can at times be diminished in severity if the individuals are protected against red and yellow, if they wear, for instance, spectacles with green lenses." Those wishing to pursue these ideas in greater depth are recommended to study the books of Faber Birren.

While most color studies have been from the psychological point of view, some doctors are beginning to realize that the eye needs moderate contrast and variety if it is to function well. Hospitals, which are rather emotive places, are choosing soothing colors for waiting rooms and wards. When one recalls the early days of grim antiseptic surroundings in hospitals and similar institutions, one is thankful that most of them, nowadays at least, make an effort toward a cheerier environment recognizing that brightness and vividness of color tend to arouse autonomic functions, blood pressure, and heart and respiration rates. Dimness and softness of color tend to have reverse effects and to invite repose; autonomic functions are retarded and there is more inner relaxation.

In surgery, the problem of glare from high-intensity lights has led to the use of turquoise and blue-green in surroundings as well as for garments; this reduces brightness in the field of view, builds up better visual contrast, and obviates the problem of the surgeon being distracted by green after-images from from blood. For patients, soft tones, not too highly reflective, are best. Ceilings should perhaps be tinted in view of the fact that some patients have to lie and gaze at them. Brilliant colors such as reds, yellows, and blues may not only prove monotonous for long-term patients, but in the case of disease such as jaundice, a yellow room would make the patient look 10 times worse! For such cases uniform lighting is important so that any change in a patient can be quickly noticed. Brighter colors in day and recreation rooms may, however, be advantageous.

In overall studies of color preferences and association of color, the three most appealing are blue, red, and green (in all their tints and variations), and the three least appealing are orange, purple, and yellow-green. Blue is better in tones of aquamarine and turquoise, as large areas of it tend to have a cold and bleak look. In short, cool, subdued colors are more suitable for chronic patients, while warm, bright colors are better for convalescent patients. Birren recommends that treatment rooms could be coral, peach, light green, or aqua, and coral for a nursery. Visitors rooms should be soft yellow, with a contrasting wall for eye interest.

Hazel Rosotti, in her book *Colour,*[8] relates how disturbed children in a residential home were asked to paint a picture. Note was taken of the dominant color in each picture, and this color was subsequently painted on the screen around individual cubicles. When the children went to bed, this seemed to settle them down for the night in a relaxed fashion. Patients at a mental hospital were found more likely to venture along a corridor painted dark purple, brown, or crimson than if it were painted a lighter color. The oppressive effect of the darker colors forced them to look for a more peaceful abode.

One of the most dramatic and controversial developments is the use of the "pink room" for calming violent people.[9] At the San Bernardino County Probation Department in California, aggressive and violent children are put in an 8 foot by 4 foot cell with one distinctive feature—it is bubble gum pink. According to Paul E. Boccumini, director of clinical services, after 10 minutes or so the children calm down, stop yelling and banging, and tend to fall asleep. What is more important, the effect lasts for some time. There are psychologists who are very skeptical of this treatment, but many authorities in the United States are experimenting with passive pink in the hope of eliminating vandalism and graffiti, while football coaches try the color in visitors' dressing rooms in the hope that their opponents will become lethargic! Whatever psychologists say, we all know that an entirely pink room does have a rather weird effect, inducing drowsiness and inertia.

Theo Gimbel, in his book *Healing Through Colour*, [10] mentions a case where a violent crowd was calmed down by Gerrard and Hessey in 1932 by using blue light. Gimbel suggests that cricket matches may be more peaceful than football because they are played in the open air rather than under arc lights. He also tells of a London exhibition in 1970 where three rooms were individually painted in black, green, and yellow. For some reason, the only room where objects were continually stolen or broken was the yellow room and from this it was concluded that people didn't like yellow. Yellow, in Gimbel's opinion, is a color that provokes violence and generates a feeling of detachment and noninvolvement. He suggests the possibility that yellow street lights may have some relevance to the incidence of crime in an area.

Schools also are trying to get away from the strictly functional image of earlier years. They tend to go in for sometimes quite exotic color schemes and brilliant murals (although whether or not this is appreciated by the pupils is another matter). What is important is the way in which the modern principles of color applied to schools will improve the scholastic performance of students, especially in their earlier years. There is always the possibility, of course, that school children who are at the receiving end of "experiments" in color may react positively simply due to the fact that interesting things are happening around them and attention is being paid to them, as has been found with factory workers in a dull environment where production shoots up when "experts"are called in to brighten up the surroundings. From the purely physical point of view, however, a background that does not harm the eyes or distract attention should be chosen—glare from too-white walls and poor visibility are to be avoided. Light colors reflect more illumination than dark ones, but too much brightness is a handicap, creating a visible "pull" away from books and tasks. Ceilings, Birren advises, should be white for good light reflection and natural wood is ideal for floors. Bright, warm colors are best for younger children and places of relaxation—soft yellow, coral, peach, and so on. The more passive effect of chartreuse (a pale yellowy-green), light green, or aqua will allow better concentration. Hence, cool colors become appropriate for upper grades and study room and libraries. End-wall color treatments are particularly appropriate in schools, where a neutral shade would be suitable for the three walls not facing the students, and a more colorful contrasting shade such as terra-cotta, old gold, avocado, turquoise, or blue breaks up the monotony by giving the classroom a different appearance from different directions. Gymnasiums and manual training and domestic science rooms are probably best in luminous tones of soft yellow, peach, and beige, while canteens and dining room should be in cheerful and "appetizing" colors such as peach, coral, rose, pumpkin, and flamingo. All obstacles should be painted bright yellow or red to draw the eye.

INNER COLOR AND NATURE

Another way in which we can experience color is subjectively, from inside ourselves. Ever since Aldous Huxley's experiments with mesca-

line, many people have tried such drugs as LSD, peyote, and even
more dangerous substances. Some of these experiments have been
conducted along scientific lines, purely for research; others have been
conducted along scientific lines, purely for research; others have been
conducted purely for self-indulgence or through misguided curiosity, without the safeguards used by doctors or those who have used
drugs traditionally as a means of spiritual-seeking. What probably
enticed most people were the descriptions given by Huxley and
others of the extraordinary visual effects, especially those involving
color. Huxley was particularly impressed by the enhanced sense of
color awareness after taking mescaline, and many people since then
have given even more titillating descriptions of the effects produced by these drugs. Strobe lamps are said to enhance one's visualization of color. From personal experience I can say that for some
hours after being subjected to a brief encounter with a strobe lamp,
my subjective visualization of color certainly seemed much easier
to achieve; however, I do not really see the point of it! Strobe lamps
can be dangerous if not properly regulated, and in the hands of the
inexperienced they can cause epileptic attacks or migraines. A less
dangerous way of subjective color experience involves the use of the
Black Box, where a person is cut off from all forms of sensory perception. After some hours spent entombed in one of these rooms,
most people experience some form of hallucination, often involving dazzling color displays. In fact, often before an attack of
epilepsy or migraine headaches the sufferer will see colored rays or
zigzag patterns before, or to the side of, his eyes. Again if one gets a
thump on the head or in the eye, a remarkable display of shooting
stars will be experienced. Colors are also experienced vividly in dreams
and meditations (this will be discussed in a later chapter).

In his book, *Access to Inner Worlds,*[11] Colin Wilson mentions a very
unusual work called *Essay on the Origin of Thought* by Jurij Moskvitin.
The author of this work describes how one day, lying in the sunlight
with eyes half-closed, he was observing the color spectrum that sometimes becomes visible when the eyelashes partly screen the eyes.
"Suddenly I became aware as if of a film in the background, a screen

or mosaic with the most strange and beautiful patterns which gave me the feeling of watching something particularly significant." He later became convinced that these patterns were made of "dancing sparks" and compared the effect to a painting by pointillist painter Signac. He began to believe that our normal vision is made up of these sparks. Colin Wilson's interpretation of Moskvitin's rather obscure ideas is that "the external world our eyes reveal to us is just a limited version of that larger inner world." In other words, "Seeing is an instantaneous act of painting, and the paintbrush is this magical rush of 'sparks' from our eyes."

Yet another way of subjectively "seeing" color is by using parts of the body other than our eyes. It has been found that many blind people develop a color sense by running their fingertips over a surface and gaining the impression that one color is warm, another cool and acid, another heavy and thick, and so on. It's quite fun to try this for yourself with color cards.

Most research on this idea seems to have been undertaken in Russia and in *Psychic Discoveries Behind the Iron Curtain,*[12] by Ostrander and Schroeder, who devoted a chapter to "Eyeless Sight." The most famous exponent of this ability is Rosa Kuleshova, who was not only able to "see" colors when blindfolded but was also able to read print and distinguish pictures simply by touching them with her hands; she said it took several hours a day of practice. Almost overnight she became a celebrity and Russians took to "the great eyeless sight fad" with immense enthusiasm. Unfortunately, the same sort of hysteria gripped the nation as metal-bending brought about in Britain in the wake of Yuri Geller and somewhat discredited the subject. In the background, however, scientists tried to uncover the mechanics of this unusual ability. It was first thought that Rosa was supersensitive to the texture of dye, but she was able, after being securely blindfolded and placed behind a thick cardboard screen, to identify red, green, and yellow even when tracing paper, cellophane, or glass covered the color sheets. They then thought she might be supersensitive to heat and so used heated plates with cool colors and vice versa; but this didn't make any difference. She was also able to identify colored liquids in a glass tube. Using both hands Rosa was able to "see" the color of anything from a tie to a postage stamp. After consulting old records, it was found that other people also had this ability. One doctor at the Nizhniy Tagil Pedagogical Institute found that about every sixth person could tell the difference between two colors after about half an hour's practice. Most people agreed that colors divide into smooth, sticky, and rough sensations—light blue is the smoothest, yellow is very slippery. Red, green, and dark blue are sticky, while violet was very sticky and rough. Not everyone "sees" color like this—Rosa herself sensed various colors as crosses, straight lines, dots, and so on.

Dr. Novomeisky, who undertook most of these experiments, believes eyeless sight has something to do with electromagnetic fields. He tried putting the color cards in an insulated tray, and his students began to react as if the color extended some way above the tray into space. Different people sensed colors at differing heights but all took similar steps up the color spectrum—for everyone, red extended highest and blue extended least. Further experiments were carried out with sightless people by beaming colored light onto their palms; eventually this was extended to the outlines of letters. Today eyeless sight is called "biointroscopy," and as further experiments are being carried out, perhaps it may develop into an ability which can be acquired by most sightless people.

The Russians say that all one's skin has seeing potential. They report trainees sensing light and color with the tongue, elbow, and nose. One wonders if this also could be extended to the senses of taste, hearing, and smell. Many claims have come out of China regarding children able to "see" with their elbows, stomachs, knees, and so forth. It is a fascinating subject but how much is due to the "experimenter effect" is open to debate. The experimenter effect is an increasingly common explanation of a phenomenon whereby the experimenter is thought to be unconsciously influencing his subjects—often the experiments in question are not able to be repeated by others.

Let us now turn from the somewhat sterile world of science to the natural everyday life around us. Many brilliant color effects in nature are not chemical in origin. The rainbow and similar manifestations—the iridescence of oil on water, soap bubbles, birds' feathers, and so forth—are phenomena of light caused by refraction, polarization, and so on. Many nonmetallic colors found in birds' wings, for example, are formed by small air bubbles in the feathers that cause white rays to split apart into their component colors. A similar process occurs through interference of light rays as they pass through the thin layers of wings of butterflies, dragonflies, and various beetles. Nothing is quite what it seems. Even the luster of mother-of-pearl is caused by light defraction. Such color manifestations from the sunrise and sunset are a result of scattered light, and heavy dust particles in the atmosphere can account for some spectacular effects. Light scattering also accounts for blue eyes, blue feathers, and the highly decorative rear end of the mandrill baboon. In fact, light scattering accounts for a lot of coloring in nature and this, as said before, can be caused by tiny air spaces. Most colors come about by absorption or selective reflection, whereby, say, a red surface absorbs most of the rays at the blue end of the spectrum and reflects back the remainder—the red!

It is therefore an interesting thought that when we are looking at a person of another color, we are really only looking at someone whose skin has the ability to absorb certain color rays and reject others. Even so, certain ailments can cause the skin to change color dramatically. Perspiration can change color under stress, as in 1709 when, the skin of an unfortunate girl turned dark and she was accused of witchcraft. In the animal world, hippopotami, for example, exude red perspiration.

Many insects, animals, fish, and reptiles change their colors according to the environment, time of year, even the time of day. Crabs and shrimps, for instance, can adapt their coloring to their environment because their skin is covered in pigment cells that are stimulated through the eyes to effect the necessary color change. Tropical fish, in particular, undergo very interesting color changes, often for no obvious reason. The chameleon is well-known for its color-changing abilities and is extremely sensitive to light (this appears to be regulated through its eyes). Many creatures use their color as defense camouflage or to disguise themselves while lying in wait for prey; others flaunt brilliant "poisonous" colors to deceive an intending predator.

Nature displays a vast ingenuity in arranging color effects: small lenslike structures in mosses make them gleam; iridescence and fluorescence in seaweed, molds, and fungi; and luminescence in the ocean (often caused by bacteria) or in such living creatures as corals. Birren tells us that much has been discovered about the luminous organs of deep-sea creatures. :Some have organs like eyes, which emit light." Nearly all deep-sea creatures are luminous or have luminous spots which are often colored—in fact, some look like crafts from outer space with rows of green, red, and orange spots. Some deep-sea creatures become luminous at mating time; others may become luminous in order to attract prey or frighten hostile predators or so that like may recognize like.

Going from the sea to the sky, the color and variety of stars seems infinite, planets and suns are quite easily identifiable as blue, red, gold, and so on. Sirius, for example, is one of the most colorful stars seen in the winter skies in the northern hemisphere, flashing and sparkling in rainbow colors. There also is the aurora, that spectacular display of dancing lights at the poles, prosaically caused by the bombardment of air by electrons and other particles that stream in from the sun in great quantity and at great speed.

In terms of color, much on our earth is affected by the time of day, season of the year, and weather conditions, when the quality of light changes dramatically from dawn to dusk. This, in turn, subtly affects all life, regulates procreation and growth, slows down and speeds up all processes in the human and nonhuman kingdoms. Even the color of soil varies tremendously according to the various minerals present in it. Stone, rock, and sand, even ordinary looking pebbles, have a beauty of their own when examined closely. Hazel Rossotti[13] tells us that some of the most beautiful colors of the mineral world are caused by optical interference. For instance, opal absorbs little visible light and is made up almost entirely of silica and water; in fact, it acts as a diffraction grating. Depending on the angle of viewing, light of one or more wavelengths is cancelled out, and thus the opal appears to change its colors continuously. Cut diamonds spread light far more effectively than a dewdrop or a glass prism because the various colors emerge at different angles according to how the diamond is faceted. Other gems owe their color to various minerals and ores present in their structure, which in turn absorb some rays and reflect others. Again, as the makers of fireworks well know, chemical elements have their characteristic fire colors—a green flame for copper and pale mauve for potassium, for example. This is evident in the variety and color of fire in all its aspects.

Thus, the four elements—earth, air, fire, and water—give us endless examples of the effect of color and the interaction of light with everything from oxygen particles to minute water bubbles. Earth has its flowers, fruits, rocks, and human and animal life in great colorful profusion; air provides us with splendid sun and sky effects, while water, ever-changing, offers an endless interplay of light and subtle color.

3

Color
in Our Living

Exterior Color

Place of Work

Most people may not think they notice the colors that assail them from all sides in their everyday environment—one's general surroundings, other people's dress, brightly colored advertisements—it all seems to pass by as a blur. But we still react fairly sharply and our eyes and bodies have registered a particular color often long before our conscious self is aware of it.

In our place of work, that environment where perforce we spend most of our days, unless we are particularly fortunate we tend to be surrounded by drab shades of beige, cream, and dirty gray. Luckily most large organizations are becoming a little more color conscious, realizing that a depressing background makes for depressed workers. Clearly, though, as action is usually required at places of work, it wouldn't do to have a soporific background and too many soft, warm lights about the place.

Much depends on the type of work to be undertaken. Color improperly applied can interfere with tasks, distract from work, and cause much eyestrain. If one is an office worker, for example, a neutral and nondistracting, cool color helps to keep the eye at a comfortable level of adjustment. The desk should also be in a neutral shade—gray, for instance, reduces the effect of blinking and thus reduces fatigue. When workers glance up their eyes should rest on a pleasing, relaxing color such as blue, green, or turquoise. Too much white causes glare and constricts pupil openings, but deep colors can open the eyes too wide and lead to eye fatigue. Soft, clear colors, with possibly a contrast wall, are best. White is very tiresome to look at if one suffers from "sleepers" in the eye—a white page such as this provides ample opportunity for them to appear. Also, in glancing from a strong color to white, one always gets a distracting afterimage. Deep or strong colors should never be put on window walls but are best placed on walls behind desks, or on walls facing people. Good colors for offices, study rooms, and fine assembly in industry are the cool hues— gray, blue, green, turquoise. There is thus less outer distraction and a person can concentrate on precision work.

On the other hand, if you work in a factory or workshop where there is much manual activity, brighter colors around the place may be more helpful. Over the last few decades most industrial plants have made a great effort to improve lighting and introduce various color schemes in the hope of inspiring their workers to greater effort. As with office workers, those workers who have to undertake intricate tasks need to rest their eyes on a pleasing, nondistracting color when they look up. Although it is impossible to enter into any great detail about color schemes for business and industrial units within the scope of this book, a few major priorities should be mentioned. In several of his books Faber Birren suggests a color scheme he has devised for factories, much of which now seems standard practice in the more advanced industrial complexes. Most suggestions are common sense—machinery should be highlighted with pale colors to reflect more light on the important parts; vivid yellow and black bands should be used to emphasize hazards and obstructions; vivid orange for acute hazards likely to cause harm or shock; brilliant green for all first aid equipment; vivid red for firefighting equipment; vivid blue as a standard caution signal; white, gray, and black for traffic control. Last, but not least, Birren recommends that corners should be painted white to discourage litter and to catch the eye of the sweeper. Many of these ideas have been adopted in railway, road, and other public service systems.

Another area in factories and offices that has long been neglected is the washroom, which is usually painted in dire shades, no doubt in the hope that one will not be tempted to linger. Since men seem to prefer blue and women prefer pink or coral, it would be appreciated by workers if these dreary places could be brightened up a little with at least a touch of these colors. Cafeterias and canteens also can be fairly dismal, and appetizing colors—the "warm" colors, or pleasantly fresh, cool hues—can help in achieving a relaxed meal break.

Shopping and Eating Out

Nowadays there is every sort of shop for every sort of customer and a subsequent thriving industry in color and decor arrangement devoted to bringing customers in. Even so, we have probably all had the experience of entering a café or shop and immediately recoiling because of the unfavorable impression it gives. Perhaps some people don't mind buying clothes in a shop where the color scheme and lighting makes them look like something out of a chamber of horrors or eating their meal in Dante's Inferno! I remember a meal in what seemed like a delightful little restaurant where the lighting was so poor that everything we ate looked dark brown. I wouldn't go there again.

Poor lighting and indifferent color schemes do not encourage people to buy, and owners of clothes and food shops may wonder why they are not doing well. Sensible shopkeepers try to align their color scheme to their wares. Most men's shops are decorated in dignified, dark, warm colors that give the impression of a discreet "men's club" atmosphere. Shopkeepers know full well that most of their customers are fairly conservative and wouldn't appreciate anything feminine or trendy. However, a different color scheme applies to women's shops, for conditioned as we are from birth to accept certain colors as feminine and others as masculine, most of us like to buy our clothes in pretty or opulent surroundings.

Unfortunately, most clothes shops and large stores don't seem to understand that a cold white light won't help their sales. Anywhere that customers have to see themselves in a mirror would fare better with warm, low-intensity lighting, similar to what is found in most of their homes. According to Birren, the most flattering background color for complexions is turquoise, ideal for clothes shops and beauty parlors. A white background tends to dull the complexion; red drains it of pinkness and lime green turns it purple! While sitting under a hairdryer in the hairdressers does tend to turn one's face puce, it's surprising the number of hairdressers who still use poor lighting and unflattering background colors.

When shopping for food we tend to have idealistic color memories, and many foods are tinted because we always remember them as more colorful than they really are. Given two jars of peas, most people will choose the tinted one. Butter is colored to give it that rich, golden dairy-fresh look; jams have to appear as if the fruit has just been picked. Some colors are "sweet" and others "savory," and if foods are colored out of context, it generally diminishes our appetite immediately. Wines are liked in golden yellow, deep red, and pink, reminding us of lush bunches of grapes hanging on the vine. Pink or blue bread would not be very popular because we have that vision of golden brown loaves made from ripened wheat. Colors such as mauve and yellow-green can cause nausea and sickness and are not very good choices for food shops or restaurants. Here again, turquoise is a good color for the display of food—meat looks redder and other foods stand out well.

Advertisers play on all these associations, suggesting to us that various foods are "harvest fresh" and bursting with natural vitamins, while in reality they are probably heavily tinted to induce just that reaction. Bright and warm colors are the appetizers and these are good in restaurants, especially those that wish to encourage people to linger; others wanting a fast-turnover of customers should go for something cooler like blue or green. The color of plates and tablecloths also plays a great part in presenting food attractively, and most pastel shades are suitable.

Home

From shopping and eating out we return to our own homes where we can express our own personalities. A few guidelines can be given for home decoration, but it is infinitely preferable to make one's own choice. It is no good to have a color scheme just because it is fashionable—you have to live with it. There are various booklets in furnishing shops that offer suggestions for particular types of rooms, although it is important that you give a room the stamp of your own personality. Many of the devised layouts in these professionally arranged rooms seem very bland or claustrophobic, with curtains and wallpaper in the same profuse pattern.

First, you have to take into account such factors as the use of the room, whether it faces a warm or cool direction, how much sun it gets, and whether you want a peaceful, relaxing room or something a little more stimulating. If you want a soothing color scheme for a bedroom for example, then pale colors, soft warm pinks or apricot, or cooler blues and greens, or mixtures of these, would be appropriate. If you want colorful curtains and cushions, then a neutral background is best; but remember that white can be tiring for the eyes. For activity rooms like the kitchen, more stimulating colors may appeal—unless, of course, you tend to be temperamental while cooking, in which case cooler hues may be very necessary!

Dark, narrow rooms need light, sunshiny colors; and while colored ceilings can be oppressive in small rooms, in a large or high room they are very helpful in bringing a ceiling "down." But don't overdo any one color. I once saw a drawing room decorated entirely in blue, with the final touch of a beautiful blue shawl flung over a grand piano. The effect was magnificent but decidedly chilly. Conversely, a room with lots of red may irritate some people or too much green may depress them. Strive for a balance of one key color with some of its complementaries in various tints and shades. Don't overdo strong colors or let yourself fall into the trap of getting together a mass of colors that go with anything—you'll end up with a sludgy beige room!

If you are outgoing, then your home will probably display bright, warm colors, perhaps with modern furniture and jazzy patterns. If you are quieter, you will probably go for a more traditional effect with cool, restrained colors. But don't try to change your nature by taking advice from others to be bolder or more subtle, otherwise you may feel unhappy with colors that are not "you." Excitable people are not necessarily better off with subdued colors, which can make them feel bottled up; likewise, quieter folk can feel very irritated in brash, trendy surroundings. Small children, who generally like bright colors, are often more tense and difficult in a too-peaceful environment. Cheerful colors relieve nervousness by creating an outward stimulus to balance the inner high spirits. However, putting a sad, depressed person in too-bright surroundings often makes them retreat even further into their shell.

We must decide for ourselves whether we prefer a bright and colorful environment or a cool and peaceful one—why not have both in your home? Just remember that warm and luminous colors—yellow, peach, and pink—tend to direct the attention outwards and increase general alertness and physical activity. They are good colors for anywhere manual tasks are performed. To some extent our color choices are conditioned by our culture and upbringing; for instance, Latin people tend to like bright, warm colors and Nordic people tend to like cool restrained colors. In the temperate zone we fall between the two and thus have plenty of scope. Some people are keen on the great outdoors and like to recreate a forest glade in their homes, with green carpets and blue ceilings, while others go for a more cozy effect, a warm "cave," conveying an impression of comfort and security. Others like strictly utilitarian bathrooms and kitchens in functional primary colors or even black and white. People of a more sybaritic disposition may prefer sea-grotto bathrooms and country kitchens out of old Provence, redolent of herbs and baking bread.

Whatever your choice, remember that colors seem more intense in large areas than small and that color cards are often very deceptive. If in doubt when covering a large area, aim for a lighter shade than the color card shows. For example, a pale luminous shade like yellow will be most deceptive on a card, but if you dilute the paint with up to 50 percent white, then the color of the card and the wall will look very much the same. If you like brilliant colors have them on one wall only (not the window end) and you won't be depriving yourself! If you prefer deep colors note that in an artificially lit room they will probably be fine during the day, but at night they have a way of crowding, causing feelings of oppression.

Clothes

The same can be said for clothes as for decorating your home—it's a matter of personal preference and common sense. There are the usual fashion tips: pale colors make large people look larger, dark colors narrow thin people down even more, bright colors "push out," and subtler shades recede. But if a large, extroverted person likes wearing bright colors, why shouldn't he or she? People won't feel happy if they force themselves into something dull and receding. We all have to wear dull clothes at times, for reasons of expediency, our work, and so on, but it shouldn't become a permanent state. If you can't afford to refurbish your wardrobe, then a bright scarf or tie will give the outside world the impression that at least you're alive and kicking! With today's fashions, of course, almost anything goes, though there are still some rather unlovely results of people adopting fashion too slavishly. Here again, however, it may be that this is the effect they want to achieve. There is plenty of scope to experiment with unusual colors, so don't be limited to the color of your eyes. Try something totally different for a change.

It is a surprising fact that while nowadays clothes are available quite cheaply, often even those who can afford better things pay little attention to color harmony in their dress, either wearing the same drab mixtures or mixing colors with no regard for a balanced effect. It makes the world a brighter place if everyone dresses a little more adventurously—and it may well affect the wearer also! I am not suggesting that we all go around as if arrayed for a wedding, but we can give a little thought as to the effect of one color against another, how they detract or add something to each other and whether the general effect is pleasing. Too many people either seem to feel that drab, dreary clothes are a mark of modest and self-effacing natures or they adopt an unhealthy "I'm drab anyway, so I'll wear drab clothes" attitude. This reveals an exhausted state of mind, rejecting color for being all too much in a complex world. A little effort to introduce some upliftment may well help the wearer immensely, for instead of being faced with their usual lackluster reflection in the mirror, their eyes will be drawn to that cheerful scarf or tie, and this will have a pleasing and cheering effect.

There are those, of course, who deliberately cultivate the Earth Mother or Son of the Soil look, forgetting that Mother Earth goes in for some fairly brilliant color effects. Punk fashions may not be to everyone's taste but no one can accuse them of being dreary. While the outside world generally judges us by our appearance, sensible folk know that this is not always an accurate assessment. Even so, the way we dress does portray something of our inward nature and our attitude to the world at large. If we dress carelessly and untidily it not only suggests something of contempt for ourselves but also for our fellow beings, unless, of course, we belong in the ranks of those elevated thinkers who consider that undue interest in dress is a sign of superficiality of mind and an excessive concern with worldly matters.

Basically, if you like quiet clothes, then be quietly elegant but wear that odd warm color sometimes. If you like very bright colors, try something subtle for a change. It might make other people look again—even if it's a mistake, at least you've registered!

INTERIOR COLOR

Color Associations

If we dislike a certain color it may be because we associate it with some unpleasant or frightening memory, something perhaps long forgotten. Old superstitions die hard; green is still considered unlucky by many people and someone "looking green" is nauseated. Green also means immaturity and naïveté, but it is usually connotations of the Fairy Folk and being *their* color that gives green its reputation of ill luck.

We may like a color in one texture or form and not in another. You might like purple velvet but detest purple cars, which brings us to "purple prose," "born in the purple," and "purple with rage," all of which have somewhat different meanings.

As said before, we associate colors with warmth and coolness, and people tend to fall into one or another of these groups. But this can be a case of our eyes deceiving us because there is no difference between, say, a red woolly vest and a blue woolly vest—the former just looks warmer. Blue seems linked with loneliness and depression—"blue-devilled," a "fit of the blues," "blues" music, and so on. Blue was worn by prostitutes and so we have "blue," implying obscenity, cancelled out with a blue pencil (an association of World War II). The German blau can also mean drunk, and it is claimed that alcohol causes visual images to become more blue and distant than normal.[1]

Even the warmer colors have their problem areas, although generally they are a little more positive. Apart from "red for danger," one "paints the town red" and has a "red-letter day" but "sees red" when annoyed. Modern associations of the "red cross" bring to mind help and assistance to victims of war and accident.

Yellow is often associated with cowardice and other undesirable attributes. Any one of these meanings could have sunk into our unconscious mind at an early age, to surface later as a "dislike."

If, therefore, you have a favorite color, or find yourself always turning to one particular color for dress or home surroundings, then the color preference guide that follows may give you some insight into the reasons for this choice (see also Figure 2). Our color preferences often change over the years and we may go through phases of wearing a particular color, say blue, at a time when we very much desire peace and stability in our lives. Before you consult the color list, however, please remember that these are only guidelines and nothing more. While some people with psychiatric problems have violent love/hate reactions to color, the majority of people tend to be less extreme. If you dislike a color intensely, it might be interesting to find out why, but it doesn't mean that you're due for a session with the nearest psychiatrist!

Figure 2: *Complementary Colors*

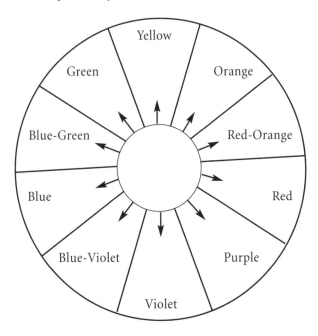

White is symbolic of purity, innocence, and naïveté. It has strong connotations of youth and freshness. A touch of white in the dress always looks fresh and attractive, and on young girls white usually looks appealing and appropriate. Certain religious groups wear white to symbolize purity of heart and a desire for simplicity or the simple life, but when it is worn continuously for reasons other than religious convictions, and by older folk, it may suggest someone who is rather immature, someone with a desire for perfection and with impossible ideals, maybe someone who is vainly trying to recapture their lost youth and freshness. Worn in conjunction with other colors, however, it shows a lively and well-balanced personality. We all need a touch of white in our lives.

Red is the color of strength, health, and vitality. It is often the color chosen by someone outgoing, aggressive, vigorous, and impulsive—

or who would like to be! It goes with an ambitious nature but those who choose it can be abrupt and crude at times, determined to get all they can out of life. They may be quick to judge people and take sides. They are usually optimistic and can't stand monotony; they are rather restless and expect to be riding high all the time. They are not usually very introspective folk and therefore not too aware of their own shortcomings. They find it hard to be objective and tend to blame others for any mishaps. If an outwardly quiet person is very fond of red, they either feel the need for the warmth, strength, and life-giving qualities of red, or they need to blanket their true feelings under a sober exterior. Generally, however, it is chosen by those with open and uncomplicated natures, with a sympathy and zest for life.

As with any color, too much red is the sign of imbalance and if you are an introspective person given to red, it might be as well to ask yourself why you need it so much.

Maroon, according to Birren's interpretation, is "passion tempered by conscience or adversity." In short, harsh experience has probably matured one into a likable and generous person. It is a favorite of those who have been somewhat battered by life but have come through. It indicates a well-disciplined "red" personality—one who has had difficult experiences and has not come through unmarked but who has grown and matured in the process.

Pink embodies the gentler qualities of red. It symbolizes love and affection without passion and in women, tends to be linked with maternal types. Someone very fond of pink desires protection, special treatment, and a sheltered life. They require affection and like to feel loved and secure. The implications of red may be frightening for them, and often the "baby pink" worn sometimes by rather large ladies may reveal a desire to be looked upon as delicate and fragile. However, it is a color with warm connotations. Those for whom it is the favorite tend to be charming and gentle, if a trifle indefinite.

Pink comes in a variety of tints from a rich strawberry to a pale apple blossom and looks lovely as a secondary in your color schemes, but too much of it gives the impression that one is living in a cloud-cuckoo land where everything is seen through rose-colored spectacles.

Orange is the color of luxury and pleasure that appeals to the flamboyant and fun-loving who like a lively social round. They may be inclined to dramatize a bit, and people notice them, but they are generally good-natured and popular. They don't care, however, for someone else hogging the limelight and may get a trifle sulky if this goes on for too long! They can be superficial, fickle, and vacillating, but on the whole they like people and have a "hail-fellow-well-met" attitude and a distinct gift of the gab. While they try hard to be agreeable, they tend not to notice the slings and arrows of misfortune, especially other people's! According to Harold Bopst,[2] orange is the color of youth, strength, fearlessness, curiosity, and restlessness. It adds stimulus to cool colors, and its complementary is blue.

Orange is one of those colors we can all do with a little of, and it adds an invigorating touch to an otherwise dull color scheme. Overall it can be rather too much, although diluted down as apricot, for example, it has enough of pink in it to curb its more exuberant qualities. In the unlikely event of someone wanting to surround themselves with orange, or always wearing it, one would think they felt a great need for the stimulating qualities of both red and yellow.

Yellow is another of the primaries and fairly popular. It is the color of happiness, wisdom, and imagination. A strong liking for yellow reveals the mentally adventurous, searching for novelty and self-fulfillment. Among their ranks are the high-minded and philosophic, especially drawn to cults and pantheistic and occult organizations. Yellow also usually goes with a sunny and shrewd personality, with a good business head and a strong sense of humor. It is the color of intellectualtity and all things to do with the mind. Yellow people are usually clear and precise thinkers who have a good opinion of their own mental capabilities and who have lofty ideals. They do at times tend to shun responsibility, preferring freedom of thought and action. They also like admiration but angle for it more subtly than red or orange. Another warm color like red, yellow has some similar attributes but on a mental level, whereas red tends to be on the physical. Both share qualities such as impatience and a mentally out-going attitude (though not so much physically for yellow—in fact, they may be rather shy). They usually have strong convictions and can be rather stubborn and opinionated. Yellow does have a strongly negative side, and when overdone it can be unpleasant. But for something or someone that needs brightening up, a dark room or a boring item of clothing, yellow in all its various applications brings a touch of sunshine and gook cheer. Not liking yellow may well point to a fear of introspection, of dipping too deeply into one's own mental depths, or of being caught up in ideas that may cause one to feel trapped or forever allied to some uncomfortable thoughts. Many people are afraid of being alone with their own thoughts, of breaking away from the conventional, or of being caught up in the swirling waters of the mind—a touch of yellow would do them good and throw a bright beam of light on hitherto unexplored regions of themselves. Its complementary color is violet.

Green is the color of harmony and balance. It symbolizes hope, renewal, and peace, and is usually liked by the gentle and sincere. They are generally frank, community-minded people, with a moral, but not prudish, approach to life. They are usually fairly sociable but prefer the quiet and peace of a country life and, in fact, sometimes prefer peace at any price, with all its negative connotations. They can be too self-effacing, modest, and patient and so often get exploited by others. They are usually refined, civilized, and reputable—but they tend to do the popular thing too often. They are often very good teachers, if a trifle garrulous.

Green can sometimes be a very depressing color and too much gives a cool and detached impression. If you find yourself continually picking out clothes in green, or always surrounding yourself with it, you may suffer from quite a high level of anxiety of which you are unaware. Green gives that feeling of everything being right in the world—the permanence and harmony of nature in an insecure and hostile environment. If you overdo it, it may be time to find out if your anxieties can be reduced and to reorganize your life upon more relaxed lines. In dress and home, try to liven up green with warmer colors in all their tints and shades—red is its complementary and something along those lines would be suitable, rather than yellow, which does not show either color to advantage.

Blue is usually regarded as everyone's favorite color, along with red. One can sink into it peacefully, feel gentled by its qualities of compassion and caring—all "mother" qualities, feminine, soft, and soothing. It is a retreat from the harsh, unkind world of everyday life. However, it is also the color of deliberation and introspection, conservatism and duty. Blue people can be rigid and self-righteous—they think their intentions are honest but they sometimes manipulate reason for their own ends. Blues like to be part of a group, where as reds have an individual and bold approach to life. Sensitive and self-controlled blues like to be admired for steady character, wisdom, and sagacity—although this is really not always apparent! Blues are good mixers, affectionate and faithful, perhaps even sentimental. They are not life's pioneers, but are cautious in word, action, and dress. They often have fixed and inflexible beliefs and are sometimes worriers—especially about what others think. Blues might be said to epitomize down-to-earth (but not in the red sense) characters who have no time for something they can't understand. Blues also have a talent for self-justification and this is where the self-righteous side comes into play. They are, however, sociable folk and loyal friends, if somewhat suspicious of strangers, especially flamboyant ones! They feel that everyone should lead an upright and sober life like themselves—at least outwardly. Being patient and persevering, they are likely to do well and make good students. They will be conscientious (usually) in their work but not inspired.

It doesn't sound as if blue is one of those colors that should be anyone's favorite, does it? But like all the others, it has its positive and negative aspects. The world would be a very sorry place without the blue of sea and sky, of flowers and streams. It is the color of the cloak of the Virgin Mary, the Mother Goddess, symbolic of all the positive feminine qualities. Excitable red people sometimes prefer blue because of its promising attributes of peace and equanimity. While weak persons crave strength, the strong often seek gentleness and kindness to complement their own lack in this regard. Relief can be found through blue, although the extrovert who prefers blue will show himself in his "true colors" before long. Its complementary color is orange, and other qualities linked with blue are serenity, dignity, spaciousness, sobriety, rest, and peace.

If you find yourself choosing blue too often, it could mean that you want to bury your head in the sand, as it were, sink into the oblivion of blue and forget the trials and tribulations of your life. A continual desire for peace and oblivion points to some problem or conflict in life, as most of us like a little excitement now and then. If at all possible blues should make an effort to be more open-minded and flexible—that nasty outside world may not be as bad as you think. Try a touch of orange to brighten yourself up!

Blue-Green is an attractive but strange mix, from the point of view of color preferences. Both Birren, Lüscher, and other researchers seem to think of it as basically a color chosen by people with a high opinion of themselves, exacting and discriminating—even fussy. They are often poised and attractive persons who inspire envy and annoyance in those who feel less well endowed. It can be a sign of those who take love rather than give it. Sensitive, intellectual, and refined, with an outer confidence and sophistication, blue-greens are also persevering and stable but rather detached. They are generally very capable and tend to reject help or guidance. It seems a rather Aquarian color—its subjects always willing to help others but in a rather detached manner. They have excellent taste, are courteous and charming but expect admiration, favor, and respect and take these for granted.

Those choosing **Turquoise** are similarly complex, imaginative, and original. They often drive themselves hard and there is occasionally quite a state of turmoil under that outwardly cool exterior.

Lavender, an offshoot of purple is a pretty color but somehow too much of it can be rather cool and offputting. It is associated with vanity, ultra femininity, and aloofness and is often chosen by the sort of person who "lives on a higher plane," who never notices anything sordid and who is always impeccable and beautifully dressed. They are on a continual quest for culture and the refined things of life, high and noble causes—provided their hands don't get dirty and nothing "earthy" is involved. All in all, perhaps a bit dainty, but you can depend on them to be charming, witty, and civilized and endowed with all the social graces. They are usually artistic (or have pretensions that way) and like to cultivate others on the same uplifted plane. They are very impressed by greatness, and there is often great determination to get one's own way. Mauve and lavender people are inclined to live in a world of fantasy, but there's a commonsense streak hidden away together with a very strong instinct for self-survival! There is often great creative talent, especially in design of various kinds—one thinks of the rather exotic male dress designer or the hostess who holds elegant little parties where all the guests are very refined and cultivated.

Lavender may be chosen by people who desire to get away from sordid conditions in their lives or who have higher aspirations than those in their present lifestyle. Its complementary is one of the variations of yellow.

Purple, a really flamboyant color, is actually not all that popular. It has connotations of mourning, solemnity, pomp, and ceremony. It is certainly not an easy color to live with in large quantities—it is very "heavy" and needs a powerful personality to carry it off well. If you really prefer purple to all other colors you may be suffering from delusions of grandeur—or maybe you really are grand! At the least it shows a strong desire to be individual—even eccentric. It is a color usually associated with the Madame Arcarti type of clairvoyant—all beads and purple plush robes. Purple people are usually fastidious, witty, and sensitive but with a strong desire to be "different." They have Jupiterian attributes and are expansive and extroverted but also highly strung, temperamental, and "artistic." Purples can also be aloof, sarcastic, and introspective when misunderstood. More interested in culture than humanity, purples often have highfalutin ideas about life. On the good side they are unconventional and tolerant, interested in philosophy and often verbose about their ideals while not actually doing anything about them. They are dignified and like to achieve a position of authority, which they regard as their natural place. They can be intellectual snobs. Bopst considers purple the color of the nucleus of all life impulses—the color of the opening bud, the first streak of dawn, and the last ray of the setting sun. He maintains that purple can produce a high state of exhilaration, but this is soon followed by an equally intense state of irritation and finally depression.

He quotes the analogy of hearing a single pleasing sound; however, pleasing in itself it cannot be endured for long.

If purple is really your color maybe you should get down from that throne once in a while and brighten up your color scheme with some variations of its complementary, yellowy-green.

Brown is the color with stamina and patience for solid and substantial people, the world's workers. We come down to earth with a bump when considering brown. Browns are usually very conscientious, dutiful, dependable, steady, and conservative. The brain may be a bit slow but the information gets there in the end. Your real brown freaks are not impulsive creatures, and they may be a bit inarticulate and tactless, but they love responsibility and can always be relied on to do that job that nobody else wants; thus, other people take advantage of them. They are salt-of-the-earth types and are usually kindly except when they come up against the world's loafers. Browns can be rather careful about their finances and don't believe in throwing good money after bad. Meanness might be an exaggeration but it has been known. They can be very obstinate in habits and convictions and don't like change. The less-brown natives are sometimes shy but warmhearted, and they like to feel needed, which may result in them always helping the underdog. They know how to strike a good bargain but don't believe in making strenuous efforts of a physical or mental nature. Their real problem is inflexibility and inability to adapt easily.

Overdoing brown, of course, means overdoing the more negative side of brown—being too plodding, dull, and inert. But brown is a very good background color that can be brightened up by more colorful accessories. It can act as a ballast, balancing out an otherwise too exotic color scheme.

If you find yourself always wearing brown, other than for reasons of expediency, then try to break away occasionally, or brighten it up with cheerful accessories—it seems to go well with most other colors especially something unusual like pink, turquoise, or apricot.

Gray is the color of caution and compromise, a balance between the extremes of black and white, a search for composure and peace without expending any inner sources of energy. Those who like gray turn away from excitement and worldly things, thus it is often a color worn by the dedicated, who will work hard without reward. It is often preferred by older people who like life to run on an even keel with few ups and downs, but when worn continually by someone young, it suggests a withdrawal from life, a renunciation of all the good things abounding in the world, and a blurring of insight, a suppression of the personality. Often grays have business ability and tend to over work. Like brown, gray is a good background color if livened up with warm and bright colors.

Black is the color of mystery! It is often worn by those who wish to give this impression, but for the truly sophisticated it is dignified and impressive, without being too showy. When dark colors are always worn it can signify the suppression of inner desires and worldly aims, suggesting hidden depths and secret longings. It is often worn by women in male-dominated countries, where it is presumably worn for "protection," but one gets the impression that such women are encouraged to fix their minds on higher things, negate their personalities, and simply exist to fill the role of wife and mother. Black can look magnificent or dowdy, depending on the wearer, but an all-black ensemble can be rather like the advertisement for "Keep Death off the Road"!

Color and Psychology

Birren gives examples of the work of various psychologists such as Felix Deutsch, Kurt Goldstein, and others too numerous to mention here.[3] From such studies it appears that to many mentally or emotionally disturbed people, especially schizophrenics, color is an unwanted intrusion in their lives, and they neither like it nor want it. On the other hand, people suffering from exhaustion or nervous breakdown show little reaction to color at all. Manic-depressives, however, delight in color (presumably on "good" days). In the Rorschach Test (the inkblot tests in black and white and color) it has been noted that introverted patients tend to reject color.

It has been found that people with anxiety states tend to have a predilection for green, with the red impulses of hatred, aggression, and sex denied. Researcher Eric P. Moss, therefore, finds it unsurprising that red is the choice of the manic and hypomanic patient, "giving the tumult of his emotions their burning and bloody expression."[4] Yellow is the color of schizophrenia—the color of the morbid mind. Whenever we observe its accumulative appearance, there is quite likely to be a deep-lying psychotic disturbance. Note the work of such artists as Van Gogh and Louis Wain (famous for his drawings of cats) which, in their latter days when both were severely mentally ill, became significantly flamelike in coloring and appearance. The depressive person paints in somber shades of dark red and black, while the manic, in his state of overexcitement, uses a lot of bright, bold color with lots of swirls and agitated lines. Painting is often very therapeutic in such cases, allowing the patient to express his feelings without having to struggle with words.

Brown relates to paranoia; blue is also associated with schizophrenia along with yellow. Under stress, people who like blue may tend to see the environment connected with their problems in some drastic manner. But blue is allied with conscious control of emotions and is the color of circumspection.

It does not follow, of course, that because we favor red or green or yellow we are suffering from any of the above conditions. Nevertheless, red is usually chosen by extroverts, and yellow is chosen by people who have an intellectual bent (although yellow is also associated with mental deficiency!).

Green is often the choice of those who are superficially intelligent, social, chatty, and with big appetites! Continual choice of green suggests escape from anxiety, sanctuary in the untroubled greenness of nature.

Narcissism is revealed by a preference for blue-green. It may indicate fastidiousness, sensitivity, and discrimination. Such people often have pronounced self-love and self-sufficiency and are difficult patients for the psychiatrist.

One of the most readable researchers on the psychological aspects of color is Dr. Max Lüscher. His book, *The Lüscher Colour Test,*[5] has been translated into English and is quite easy for the intelligent layman to grasp. Precise instructions are given for assessing one's own personality as well as the personalities of others. As with all these "methods," caution should be exercised, as they are not meant to be used as party games.

Dr. Lüscher's method entails choosing eight colors in order of preference. The test is based on the arrangement of these eight colors and their relationship to one another. If one chooses honestly, the ways in which combinations work out (in terms of personality assessment) can be quite a blow to one's ego. As with all such tests, once you know roughly the "correct" answers, it becomes rather difficult to be objective and not cheat!

Without giving away too much of the test, it is interesting to compare Dr. Lüscher's findings with those of other researchers. I tend to find these tests a little negative at times, because it seems that whatever you choose, you can't win. They were presumably first devised for people with problems, and we must keep this in mind and not despair if our personalities are less than perfect.

Dr. Lüscher's color cards (in the book version) are not all true primaries—the red is orange-red; the blue is dark blue; the green has a lot of blue in it; the violet has a lot of red; and the brown is a rather unattractive shade. Yellow is the only true primary. Since none of the colors are, to my mind, particularly attractive, this may ensure that the person choosing the cards is more honest. You can check these color meanings against those given earlier—in many instances there certainly seems to be a correlation.

Red is assigned most of the qualities already outlined in earlier pages. It is "impulse will-to-win and all forms of vitality and power from sexual potency to revolutionary transformation." Thus, a rejected red (placed in a negative position on the test layout) often signifies physical and nervous exhaustion, with its accompanying loss of potency or sexual desire or possible heart or other disorders. Those for whom red occupies a prominent place are seeking experience and fullness of life and often throw themselves into activities that can be overexaggerated—but this will be mitigated or confirmed by the color that accompanies red in the test. All in all, most researchers seem to be in agreement as to the qualities of red. Whoever places red in the "rejected" position is already overstimulated to the point where such a color irritates because of the intensity of his problems, which may appear insoluble or overdemanding. He thus throws out anything suggestive of further stress.

Blue is often put in a position where it compensates for rejected red. These two colors are often aligned where business anxieties and possible heart disease are present, and, in fact, Dr. Lüscher regards them as an excellent early warning sign. Blue thus represents complete calm. Contemplation of this color has a pacifying effect on the nervous system and, as other researchers have found, blood pressure, pulse, and respiration are all reduced, although according to Birren this is only a temporary effect because the condition reverts to an even more serious degree than the original condition. Dark blue also represents contentment and fulfillment, "truth and trust, love and dedication, surrender and devotion, representing traditional and eternal values." When this color is given priority, there is a great need for rest and relaxation and the chance to recover. Blues want a calm and orderly existence, free from contention. When chosen for a position standing on its own, as it were, and not "compensating," blue implies "quietness of spirit, calmness of manner . . . and integrity."

However, when blue is rejected it can be an indication of anxiety over business and personal relationships, probably caused by too exacting standards of perfection. There is the wish to sever ties because of these standards and, in turn, this causes restlessness and mental turmoil. It may become difficult to concentrate and may lead to disturbance of the nervous system. Sometimes red is put in a compensatory position, suggesting that the sufferer will make dramatic efforts for emotional fulfillment, either perhaps through promiscuous behavior or through some dangerous or adventurous activity such as mountain climbing or car racing. I find it hard to believe that all such enthusiasts are compensating for some great lack in their emotional makeup, however.

Green is also sometimes chosen as a compensation for rejected blue, and this suggests a proud and rebellious demand for independence.

The green in this test has more blue than yellow, thus becoming blue-green, the color of the ego. Therefore, someone who puts this color in a prominent position places a high value on the "I," his own self-awareness and self-affirmation. If this is your most favored color, it reveals, subject to its companion colors, a desire to increase self-assertiveness. You may have a somewhat idealized picture of yourself and expect others to recognize this also. Greens are proud and unchanging and very aware of their egos. Loss of face for greens often results in ulcers and digestive and stomach upsets. This color does, of course, have a positive side—its adherents are often forced to find expression in a quest for better conditions, improved health, and so on, and here we have the reformer. Unfortunately, greens tend to moralize to others and put themselves on a pedestal. Greens like to impress and would rather be admired than loved. Those who reject green and place it in a weak position also want these things but feel unable to achieve them and, therefore, suffer from a sense of pressure, sometimes exploding outwardly as a chest or heart complaint. Rejected green therefore means, according to Dr. Lüscher, "anxiety to liberate himself from the tensions imposed by non-recognition." Extreme cases are those unhappy folks who are so stubborn and self-opinionated that they are their own worst enemies.

Blue is often chosen as compensation (that is, put in the place a healthy green would normally occupy) because effort is no longer required; red compensation reveals itself in loss of self-control and impatience. Green in a "normal" position in the test is, of course, part of a natural urge we all have to express ourselves and be recognized by our fellows.

Yellow is the only true primary used in the test. It indicates qualities of expansiveness and relaxation. Although yellow also increases blood pressure, pulse, and respiration rates, it does not do so with the consistency of red. Yellow corresponds to sunlight, cheerfulness, and happiness, but it has a somewhat unstable and uncertain quality—rather Mercurial, in fact. If yellow is a first choice, it shows the desire for release and the hope of better things to come. When it occupies a major position, there is not only a great desire to escape from present conditions but a desire for change for the sake of change. If, as Dr. Lüscher says, green is "persistence and tension," yellow is "change and relaxation." If yellow is rejected, then hopes have been dashed with a resultant inner turmoil. This may result in irritability, depression, and often hopelessness. Blue is sometimes chosen instead and shows a need to hang on to the familiar and safe. If green is chosen, there may be efforts to compensate by striving after prestige and position. Unhappy yellows can have problems with the sympathetic and parasympathetic nervous systems. Yellow is usually preferred by people of an intellectual bent—but it is as well to remember that it is also associated with mental deficiency! Its rejection may be indicative of a dislike of probing too deeply into one's own mental processes and inner feelings.

Violet is a very red-blue mix that tends to fall into the category mentioned in the previous list of colors, that of the fantasy world. Those who put this particular violet in a prominent place want magic and glamour for themselves as well as others. While this may indicate some immaturity, the world would be a duller place if there were no violet people. There is a quality of unreality and wish fulfillment in the makeup of those whose main choice is violet, however, it is often chosen by the naïve and unsophisticated. Glandular and hormonal activity during pregnancy may result in a temporary preference for violet, and this also sometimes applies to people with a thyroid problem. Again, to those suffering from emotional insecurity, violet suggests a magical world where everything comes right in the end. The true violet type is sensitive and charming, often casts a spell over themselves and others, but does not want responsibility.

Brown is a dark yellow-red. Those who choose it for a major position are emphasizing the body's sensory condition. Brown indicates physical sensation and, depending where it is placed, can reveal a degree of physical discomfort. The rootless and homeless often make brown their first choice because it suggests security and ease, a place of one's own. It can indicate a need for physical ease or release from some painful or uncomfortable condition such as illness; or it can indicate a state of conflict and unsolvable problems. When brown is rejected, physical comfort is seen as a weakness revealing the "cold-baths-and-hair-shirt" type of person. When the body is denied in one way, however, it will retaliate in another, probably with some form of compulsive behavior. One is reminded of some of the early saints who were always battling with unseemly visions! In a normal position brown simply reveals the average person's desire for reasonable comfort and home and security.

Gray is the most neutral color of all, neither dark nor light. It represents a sort of no-man's-land, an area of separation between two zones. Chosen first, it indicates that the chooser wants to wall everything off and be uncommitted and uninvolved in anything. Whatever color follows usually points to an unadmitted desire represented by that choice.

Gray is, however, part of our normal makeup, and those who reject it in an equally strong fashion may try to involve themselves in too much, becoming tiresome meddlers who are anxious to miss nothing. Gray boxed in by two colors reveals a desire only to experience through the qualities of the first and to block off the second.

Gray in a prominent place in the test suggests self-deception and can be descriptive of people who are often powerful in business and industry—another urge psychologists suggest may be the result of a desire to escape from some unwarrantable anxiety!

Black expresses the idea of nothingness and extinction, renunciation and surrender. Whoever chooses black as a first choice wants to renounce everything as a protest against existing conditions. If red follows, for instance, then exaggerated desires may compensate for all that is deficient; if blue follows, then complete tranquility and harmony are expected to restore things to rights; if yellow follows, then some sudden change of course (or a miracle) is expected to end one's troubles. In the "normal" position black indicates the usual human desire not to have to relinquish anything and to be in control of one's life.

From these descriptions it can be seen that there are many tieups between Dr. Lüscher's findings and the findings of other researchers. The question of why certain colors correspond as they do to certain characteristics in our personalities is intriguing. To answer this question we can only return to the first chapter where, in the comparatively short history of humankind, colors and their associations were firmly imprinted on the collective mind: red correlates with heat, blood, life, and danger; blue, with sky,heaven, peace, mother; green, with growth (and decay); yellow, with sun, warmth, happiness; white, with purity, cleanliness, perfection; black, with mystery, death, annihilation. Many more subtle colors and qualities have arisen since those early days, but they all stem from the basic primaries.

Most people use a mixture of colors for personal use, but since all of us have a few quirks here and there in our personalities, it might be a useful exercise to investigate these. Tests like Dr. Lüscher's may be helpful, although it seems to be forgotten that most of us would never do anything if it were not for hidden urges and inner stresses driving us to take some drastic action. It is only when these stresses become unbearable, or when we can see no way out, that these tests are truly valuable.

4
Color
in Our Being

Whether the aura actually exists or not is still a matter of controversy between those who claim to see it and measure it and those who can't. For the purposes of this chapter, it will be simpler to assume that it exists and, for those unhappy with this assumption, a perusal of the works of Professor Harold Saxton Burr and Dr. Walter J. Kilner is recommended (see Further Reading).

The aura (from the Greek word *avra* meaning "breeze") is not a modern phenomenon dreamed up by psychics and mystics. Our ancestors knew all about auras, and from very early times artists have depicted them around the heads of saints and other holy persons. It was hardly likely that such a thought would have arisen without some basis in fact. Words such as halo, nimbus, aureole, and glory are descriptive of various parts of the aura—a "glory," for instance, is described as "a circle of rays surrounding the head of a saint" and an aureole is the radiance surrounding the entire body.

People of psychic sensitivity have often described a radiance surrounding not only saintly people but also ordinary folks. In the Bible, for example, Moses' face, when he came down from the mountain, shone so that "they were afraid to come nigh him."[1]

Not only human beings, but every creature and everything in nature appears to be surrounded by a radiance, ranging from the faint hazy outline to be seen around a stone to the rather larger aura of a tree. We know that every living thing gives off various electrical and other emanations—generally we can't see them, but they can be sensed and recorded by delicate instruments as well as by sensitive people, in fact, people are far more sensitive than any instrument. If we could see ourselves for the swirling mass of atoms that we are, it would be very difficult for us to regard ourselves as "solid bodies" thereafter.

Since the advent of Kirlian photography there has been a great deal more interest shown in the aura. Unfortunately, many people have made the mistake of equating the aura with the rays shown in the photographs. While they are somewhat similar in appearance to auric rays, it is probable that these rays have more of a link with electrical emanations from the body. They are certainly not the same thing as the human aura, unless one regards them as the part of it nearest to the physical body. The aura itself is much larger and more finely constituted; it can nevertheless be seen and felt by those who are sensitive enough to do so. After a little practice, most people can see the basic auric outline, but anything further than that usually requires some degree of clairvoyant sight.

To catch a glimpse of the average aura can be difficult unless there is something noteworthy about it. Auras vary considerably in density and structure, and even those who can normally see them are not always able to do so. That part of the aura closest to the physical body manifests itself as a narrow band of transparent light, sometimes a misty white, about a half-inch wide. From this the aura can expand to anything from two feet wide or even much larger, depending on the individual. Within this auric body the fluctuating colors that give it its identity can be seen.

For basic purposes, the aura of humans can be divided into three separate parts, corresponding to the basic "bodies" which reside in and around the physical vehicle. These parts comprise (1) the Etheric or Vital body, which is closest to the physical and is said to leave the body in sleep or unconsciousnes; (2) the Astral (this term can be confusing as it sometimes refers to the Etheric, depending on your school of thought) or Emotional body, which supplies most of the auric coloring; and (3) the Mental body, which the intellect and all its attributes.

The aura of women is usually seen more easily than that of men, which may be because they have more developed emotional bodies and they are more at ease in this mode of expression than men, who tend to pride themselves on being rationalistic, thinking individuals, thus restricting their emotional expression. Beyond the three levels there are even more subtle "bodies" of varying degrees of spirituality, and their colors are usually only briefly glimpsed.

To "see" an aura is to some extent an acquired knack (which is easier than people think), and you may have been aware of them for years without realizing it. The first essential is to be relaxed. Look slightly above and beyond the head of your subject, gazing into infinity. Don't try too hard or it will just elude you. A neutral background with no distracting colors is best, although some people prefer dark background. Stand your subject against a plain door or curtain and stand at least 10 feet away from them. Even against a colored background, the colors will sometimes be strong enough to override it. You can practice with nonhumans—animals, plants, and trees. You may not succeed for some time, but after a while most people are able to see the faint band of mist closest to the physical body.

Naturally there are various pitfalls to avoid when "looking" in this way. The most obvious is visual aberration. Our eyes play many tricks on us, and we have to be very honest with ourselves about what we think we are seeing. One of the main problems is eye fatigue. When the eyes become tired they tend to see a bluish green haze around the object of vision—you can experiment and see if this happens in your case. Similarly, complementary color effects can be misleading—someone wearing bright red will appear to have a green aura; likewise, if they are wearing a blue hat or have orange hair, the complementary color will comprise the aura. Only practice, and comparing notes with other sensitives, will give you the experience and confidence that what you are seeing is definitely the aura. Get acquainted with some of the tricks your eyes can play; then you should be able to sort the wheat from the chaff.

Do not lose heart, however, if you cannot see anything—you can sense auric colors by mentally tuning into your subject. It is best to begin with a practical exercise. Engage the help of a cooperative friend and seat him or her in a chair. Then hold your hands a few inches away from your friend's head and try to sense any radiations within this area. You will first become conscious of waves of bodily warmth— the head gives off quite a bit of heat. Then, perhaps if your friend is tense and unrelaxed, you will begin to sense this as a kind of vibra- tion coming from them. Slowly withdraw your hands until you reach a point where this tension appears to cease—this could be the limits of the "astral" body aura. Try to remain in a relaxed state yourself during this procedure so you can then focus your mind on the thought of auric colors, waiting to see if any specific colors relating to the sub- ject appear in your mind. This is more difficult and takes some prac- tice. Later, you should be able to look at a person, mentally tune in, and receive a color impression of their aura. This is not telepathy or an attempt to pick up their thoughts—it is a procedure that we all unconsciously use during our daily life, a continual assessment of those around us. Test the auras of as many different people as you can, and you will begin to get a general idea of how much they can vary in breadth and density. Some will feel "all over the place" and very thin or diffuse; others will be too tight, compact, and withdrawn; but the majority will have a fairly normal aura, between 18 inches and 2 feet in depth, surrounding their head and body in a generally ovoid shape. "Cold spots" or unusual emanations in the aura can be signs of damage or breaks and these will be dealt with in a later chapter. The aura is a very important protective mechanism which must be treated with the same respect as one treats the physical body.

Our auras fulfill a very important task. They protect us from a variety of subtle and not-so-subtle energies—emanations from var- ious sources, thought forms, disease organisms, and minor bumps and bruises—in much the same way that the physical skin protects the inner organs and skeleton structure of the body. In shamanistic teachings, such as those described in the books of Carlos Castaneda and Max Freedom Long (see Further Reading), the auric field is described as a mass of fine fibers standing out at right angles to the body. Depending on one's state of health and personal power, these fibers can be extended indefinitely, especially from the solar plexus and other chakric areas, for the purposes of telepathic contact, telekinesis (moving objects without any apparent means of doing so), clairvoyance, and most other paranormal abilities. In some cases of poltergeist activity, the instigator is no doubt unconsciously using personal energy through the medium of the auric rays. A ray, or fiber, can be extended to an object or another person for any variety of reasons. A good example of the auric energy being used for personal objectives is in one of Carlos Castaneda's books,[2] where the shaman Genaro manages to attach himself to rocks overhanging a waterfall by means of auric fibers. He is then able to take incredible leaps from rock to rock by these "tentacles," which keep him in place as securely as a fly on the ceiling.

It is also possible, in a more modest way, to divine the strength or weakness of people's auras. There is a distinct resistance when one comes up against a very strong auric field. Large and formidable people have an aura one can almost bounce off! It is no wonder that kings were always credited with so much personal power. Consider someone like Henry VIII, who, besides being physically large, had the authority of kingship behind him, giving a double boost to a no doubt powerful personality. There is the story of the Egyptian king who accidentally touched one of his courtiers with his staff. The poor man was convinced he would die on the spot because of the royal power; however, the pharaoh was concerned and spoke kindly to him, thus restoring him to normal.

We are making auric contacts all the time—some are very minor but others form very strong bonds indeed. Not all of these are beneficial, of course, but they are there just the same. We constantly monitor other people's auras and they, our's. Some people we do not care for and withdraw protectively into our own shell; others we respond to and feel in harmony with, and we are drawn automatically to such persons.

It is very important that the auric field be as strong as we can make it (ways to do this will be more fully described in the last chapter). Basically, it is simply a matter of thinking about the auric field and trying to imagine it surrounding the body, rather like a protective force field around a spacecraft or an atmosphere around a planet. The more one thinks about it in this manner, the stronger it becomes. There are, of course, the apocryphal stories of adepts with such strong auras that bullets bounce off them!

Very gifted clairvoyants can study an individual's aura to the extent that they can diagnose illness and winkle out one's character secrets. To such people we are going about with our lights "fully on," as easily readable as a book. Fortunately for our peace of mind, there are not too many who are able to "see" to this extent, but even if you never succeed in seeing or sensing colors you can gain a general impression of the state of a particular aura. There seems to be a brightness around some people; a dark cloud around others. Mostly we register these impressions without really thinking about them. Next time you feel something of this sort, try to analyze exactly what gives this impression—is it the facial expression, the stance of the physical form, or something beyond them both?

From Paracelsus to Mesmer, and from Mesmer to the present day, many people with a scientific and intellectual bent have endeavored to investigate the aura. One of the most widely quoted is Dr. Walter J. Kilner, medical electrician at St. Thomas's Hospital in London. In his book *The Human Atmosphere*, Dr. Kilner described a method involving a glass screen incorporating a cyanine dye, through which the human aura could be perceived. He maintained that every human body was surrounded by an emanation extending some 18 inches to 2 feet in all directions, ovoid in shape. This varied slightly from day to day and became more difficult to see during illness. In the revised version of the book, *The Human Aura,* Dr. Kilner, seemed of the opinion that the aura one was dealing with was an ultraviolet phenomenon. He noted that some women had the ability to change their auric colors at will. His book describes in great detail the diagnosis of auric fields in humans, although his diagnoses were mostly ignored by the medical profession. Many clairvoyants also dispute that the aura can actually be seen through Kilner screens and maintain that you have to be clairvoyant anyway to be able to see it and that Dr. Kilner therefore must have been clairvoyant himself. Not everyone can see an aura when looking through Kilner screens, and they may well be just a psychological prop. Kilner goggles are still available for those who wish to experiment with his methods, although it is preferable to try to see the aura without such aids. Further work in this field has been carried out by Henry Boddington, who actually devised the goggles and fitted them with double glasses between which the dye solution could be placed. Dr. Kilner was able to diagnose ailments and injuries through his method of auric viewing in much the same way as diagnoses are made from Kirlian photography nowadays,[3] possibly here again some degree of clairvoyance is involved.

Whatever your method of registering auric colors, the following notes may give you some hints on diagnosis. This is a very individual matter and should only be regarded as a guide. You may find that you will need to modify or adapt some of these interpretations according to your own findings, but on a very general basis they provide a fairly accurate framework. The main colors of the aura are those of the rainbow; they overlap at times with color interpretation in other fields.

Many color therapists work in accordance with the "vibratory rays of the universe" and S. J. Ouseley, in his informative little book *The Science of the Aura,*[4] interprets the seven color rays as follows.

Violet—spiritual power
Indigo—intuition
Blue—inspiration
Green—energy
Yellow—wisdom
Orange—health
Red—life

We can see the extent to which they fit in with color interpretations in earlier chapters. It is too general an assessment for auric diagnosis, but it is nevertheless a useful guide.

Let us commence at the most physical level—the color of life. To the finer sight there will be many graduations of hue, in varying degrees of clarity; these are interpreted through experience and, in fact, may take many years of practice to achieve.

Red in the aura, if clear and bright, reveals an abundance of vitality, sexual power, and an active, outgoing, generous, and possibly materialistic nature. Red is usually not the main color and may only appear temporarily, depending on the mood of the subject and whether they are in some state of excitation, such as anger, desire, and so on. A muddy or dark red denotes negative emotions such as hate, malice, and other destructive passions. Combined with black, red suggests very unpleasant characteristics. The visually sensitive can literally see red sparks coming out of an angry person's head, but it is only a temporary effect and can cause the head aura to open, resulting in a headache or feeling of depletion. A healthy red now and then, as with everything else, means that we are alive and kicking.

Blue-reds and orange-reds are obviously diluted reds and correspondingly affected by their companion color. A lovely rosy pink is usually associated with unselfish love, while the presence of a dull brownish gray could indicate that selfishness of some kind has crept in. There are subtler variations of red, but interpretation of the comes best with experience. Not many are able to tune in so finely.

Orange is also regarded as a rather worldly and materialistic color to have in the aura, but again it depends on the actual hue or shade. A muddy orange can indicate selfishness, an urge "to get there first," pride, and obstinacy. A clear orange, however, while of a material quality, shows normal ambition and perhaps denotes the down-to-earth person with little time for the fantastic. A pleasing apricot blends orange and pink for the kindly, commonsensical, well-balanced type of person. Again it is a sign of energy—physical vitality combined with intellectual activity (red and yellow)—but if dominating the aura, it leaves out the softening qualities of blue and pink. Dominant orange is usually the sign of an ambitious, worldly sort of person, usually fairly healthy and not given to too much introspection.

Yellow represents mental activity and can be noted in most auras when the subject is concentrating, reading, or writing or engaged in any other left-brain activity. Unless one is of the predominantly thinker type of person, yellow tends to come and go. A good yellow is an excellent color to have in the aura and it sometimes brightens into gold if the person's thinking is on a highly spiritual level. Maybe next time the vicar gives a particularly good sermon it might be worthwhile to take a look at his aura! Dingy yellows are suspect, often indicating suspicion and jealousy, clouded thinking, or at least aimless dreaming. Good yellow aura people are usually bright and cheerful, capable, and resourceful, but as said, yellow appears in most auras from time to time.

Green, with the exception of the darker shades, is usually a good color to have in the aura, but because it is the "energy" color it can also indicate depletion. I remember an occasion when a friend was giving a talk and several people present, who normally "never saw anything," noted a brightish green aura around her. Normally this lady had a brilliantly colored aura with pink, yellow, and blue intermingling, so the contrast was extreme. She had on this occasion just recovered from the flu and her energy level was very low.

Some sensitives consider a light green in the aura to denote healing ability. Other schools of thought hold that mid-green indicates adaptability and versatility (though this depends on your personal interpretation of mid-green); clear green indicates sympathy, while the darker shades suggest treachery and deceit. Too much green, as in other areas, can give a rather negative feeling of detachment and noncommitment. Green and blue combined, to my mind, always indicates intuition or at least great sensitivity.

Blue has many aspects and nearly all are indicative of positive qualities—integrity, sincerity, a strong sense of the religious, inspiration, compassion, and kindliness. As the intensity of blue deepens, the above-mentioned qualities are enhanced. Indigo, for instance, is said to show a high degree of spirituality, while paler hues suggest such qualities as self-reliance and idealism. Most people's auras have a fair amount of blue in them, and while its absence does not mean that they do not manifest any of the above qualities, it probably indicates that they are on a more mental or physical level, according to whether the predominant color is yellow or red. The "true-blue" personality is usually emotionally well-developed and more of a "feeling" type of individual. Again, muddied colors of any sort indicate a lessening of the positive qualities, a clouding and disruption of their true function.

Violet is the color of cosmic consciousness, the color that indicates the free-ranging mind able to consider life and the universe without dogmatism, able to take past and future in its scope, with an awareness that life is eternal and forever evolving.

This color is rarely seen to dominate an aura and is usually only noted in the outer fringes as an extension of the more spiritual auric bodies. Many New Age people have this color in their auras, thus reflecting the awareness and idealism of the coming Aquarian epoch.

Gray, as sometimes seen in all-gray auras, doesn't necessarily mean the subject is depressed. But certainly it doesn't denote very exciting qualities for those who have it in their auras, and they are likely to be very conventional, formal, and rather unadventurous, to say the least. Gray indicates a lack of imagination, although such people are often very good organizers. They are persistent and plodding and often described as loners or oddballs. Darker shades of gray can be attributed to severe depression or at least a very negative attitude toward life. Maybe we all get a bit gray at times but it shouldn't be a permanent state.

Black is not a good color to have in the aura. Any auras showing quantities of black should be regarded as having extremely negative aspects. Fortunately, the truly black aura is very rare; most people have some redeeming quality to their personalities. However, if it appears in combination with another color, then that color will indicate the direction of the specific negative quality in question. If mixed with red, for instance, which is the worst possible combination, it indicates hatred, cruelty, and the basest of evil desires. Such people are too dangerous to get involved with, and on such an occasion it might be advisable not to stop and examine their auras too closely but to get out while the going's good.! A black and yellow aura would indicate an evil genius of the "thinking" variety. Even so, such people may have redeeming qualities, able to justify their evil acts to themselves on a purely mental level. After all, even some of the Nazi war criminals were known to have been affectionate fathers and husbands. A black and green aura could indicate treachery, envy of the worst kind, or avarice—or possibly some severe health problem. A blackness in a specific part of the aura often points to a physical disorder of some nature, or it can indicate an "entity" or "thought form" caught up in the auric field. Any blackness at all in the aura of a living person, or an entity from some other level of being, is to be regarded with extreme caution.

Silver is considered a mercurial and rather volatile color in the aura and is usually associated with lively but rather unreliable people who perhaps have streaks of brilliance now and then. This color generally emanates from the "mental" body and therefore has all the detachment and superficiality that this might imply. Silver can sometimes be associated with excessive refinement of mind and attitudes—the "higher plane" dwellers who tend to be a bit difficult to live up to.

Pink is a lovely color to have in the aura, denoting love and affection, kindness and gentleness. Too much may indicate the "rose-colored-spectacles" type of person, but they are usually warm and responsive people who are rarely aggressive or overwhelming in any way. A fair leavening of pink in the aura makes up for a lot of deficiencies and shows a nice balance when mixed with any of the other positive colors.

Brown in the aura is said to indicate a very down-to-earth attitude, an aptitude for organization, and a materialistic approach to life. It is the color of the conventional, closed mind, with little emotion but a desire to dominate. It is not a happy color to have in large amounts, but the typical brown aura would probably be so withdrawn and uptight that it would be rather difficult to see it anyway.

White is an interesting color to have in the aura, although again this is subject to personal interpretation. In the experience of my own particular "school," white in the aura has come to be regarded as a very useful indication of the type of person who is a "transmitter" rather than a "receiver." Such people succeed in sending out telepathic impressions and healing thoughts and possibly have the ability to manipulate various levels of energy rather than be manipulated by them. It suggests a positive type of mind, not too influenced by outside impressions. Medical people, exorcists, teachers of various kinds, and all who have to deal with situations where a detached but compassionate attitude is necessary, probably tend to have a certain amount of white in their auras. Mixed with the blue-green of intuition, it makes for a formidable personality (in the psychic sense) who can combine all these qualities and receive impressions on an emotional level but be well able to evaluate them without getting too involved. Furthermore, they can coolly formulate a solution and apply it in a positive and directive manner. White often indicates a good supply of psychic energy.

It must be remembered that the aura is constantly fluctuating according to our moods and emotions and reflects our state of health on a physical level. It is our own personal aurora and reacts constantly to outside stimuli, much in the way that the earth's aurora is affected by particle streams from the sun, solar winds, and distant stars and planets. Unpleasant noise affects it adversely, causing it to constantly flicker. If one is sufficiently relaxed, however, even a road drill can be regarded with equilibrium! Sudden and severe shocks of various kinds can cause the aura to expand, become displaced, or even "break" in places, leaving the possessor unprotected and at the mercy of whatever happens to be passing at the time. Excessive sunbathing can be harmful for the aura, causing it to expand and become very diffuse. If you have noticed a feeling of weakness after prolonged sunbathing, it is sensible to try to restore the aura to its normal condition by visualizing it very strongly around yourself. Excessive drink has a somewhat similar effect, except that often the Etheric body is put completely out of alignment, resulting in an unpleasant feeling of disassociation. Drugs (narcotics) can severely damage the aura by forcing the mental bodies to "open out" in an unnatural manner and by leaving the physical body unprotected and vulnerable to negative influences and physical intruders such as germs, viruses, and so forth.

The effect all this has on the colors of the aura can well be imagined. Sometimes permanent damage results, with a weakness in the aura that has to be continually patched up. Such weaknesses can also be caused by illness or some traumatic experience in life, although in these latter cases a good healer may be able to repair the damage.

DREAMS

One of the internal manifestations of color is experienced in dreams. Much of the time, from those dreams we remember, we have monochrome or black and white dreams; but now and then we will have a dream with outstandingly vivid coloring. This may be, on the physical level, the result of chemical or electrical interactions within the brain; on another level, it may be something to do with our innate ability to visualize color. Whatever the reason, it is interesting to include symbolic color along with normal dream interpretation. Jeremy Taylor, in his book *Dream Work*,[5] puts forward the intriguing idea that people dream in color most of the time, but that most often women recall color because they have a general tendency to pay conscious attention to the realms of feeling "and to the visual and aesthetic impact of waking life." He also believes that color in dreams depends very much on our own emotional life and that red is usually the first color detected in dream recall because it is the color associated with the most basic and strongest emotions—rage, lust, love, and so forth.

According to one scientific experiment,[6] the colors most frequently seen in dreams are in the red and orange areas. This would fit with Jeremy Taylor's point that red is the first color recalled after black and white. Purples, blues, and blue-green were mostly absent. Six male observers were used in this experiment, all of whom had normal color vision. Their dreams were recorded over a period of five months. Immediately after waking they were required to identify, on a color atlas, any colors seen in their dreams. The experiment does not really seem broad enough in scope or duration to be the final word on dream color, and other research has revealed a wide discrepancy in the figures quoted. Using female subjects may reveal an entirely different pattern of dream color. Results from another survey mentioned in the same article indicate that 51% of men and only 31% of women never have, or never remember, color dreams, suggesting that dream recall is far greater for women. All that being said, inquiries among one's friends and acquaintances usually reveal that someone has had dreams involving color—and not only red. It may be useful to briefly consider how we can incorporate these colors into our normal dream interpretations. The colors can be interpreted very much along the lines already described, but a brief résumé may be helpful to qualify your interpretation according to the further content of the dream.

Red can represent, as discussed, passion, anger, strong feelings of various kinds, warmth, life, and vitality, depending on other aspects of the dream. Blood and fire are often seen in dreams, and the latter is sometimes indicative of a situation likely to become out of control if not carefully watched. Blood is life, and, depending on the content of the dream, it can be positive or negative. Red can, of course, appear in other guises—clothes, hair, sky, and so on. Most of us tend to associate red with some kind of danger or excitement, and it can thus suggest covert desires or a warning of some kind. You have to use your own common sense here. Obviously a cozy little fire would not have the same connotations as a roaring conflagration—the former suggests that a certain situation or project is steadily under way and the latter, that it is likely to get entirely out of hand. The qualities of fire—volatility, instability, but also vitality and potentiality—all add significance to dream material.

Orange is a muted form of red, so one would not allot such strong attributes to it as those of red. Orange is health, enthusiasm, and youthfulness and would seem to add a very positive quality to a dream, but here again it must be set against the general tone and feeling of the dream. We associate orange with the sun and with cheerfulness but without the fierce heat of red—a mixture of vitality and wisdom.

Yellow in dreams is another very positive color, depending on the dream scenario. It can stand for wisdom, particularly if a dream person appears dressed in yellow or gold which could represent an inner guide or some wiser aspect of ourselves. Here again common sense must be used in assessing the possibilities of a particular dream. A field of yellow wheat, for example, would appear to show that a very satisfactory outcome of something long planned is coming to fruition and that all is proceeding well; but a yellow desert scene would suggest quite the opposite. Yellow is, on the whole, a positive color, indicative of wisdom, clarity, and light.

Green in dreams is very much a symbol of life, fertility, and creativity. A lush green field of grass, compared with a few tufts in a stony landscape, speaks of at least inner vitality and the possibility of further growth with subsequent harvest. As in other areas of color interpretation, a murky or disturbed green suggests an impairment of this happy situation. Generally speaking, green is a positive color suggesting that one's life is full of energy and creativity.

Blue is said to be rarely seen in dreams, but this may be just poor recall. It is a quieter color and may not be so easy to remember. It represents spirituality, cosmic energy, and various emotional levels, depending on the content of the dream. In one sense, to see a blue sky or a blue sea could mean that one is simply reproducing an everyday factual scene—or it could mean much more. Blue, when associated with water, has emotional implications, and, as with fire, the difference between a small, still pool and a raging torrent is enormous. In the former case it suggests a need or desire for quiet contemplation; in the latter case it suggests emotions out of control, with the dreamer in danger of being swept along by overwhelming feelings. The added coloration of blue adds intensity to such dreams. Blue sky, however, gives a more tranquil, spiritual feeling to a dream, a reaching up, a striving toward the heavens. The qualities of air are lighter and more exhilarating and detached than those of water. Blue added to an otherwise drab scene could point to a positive and spiritual uplift which would improve an inert phase in one's life. If blue appears in other ways—in clothes, eyes, and so on—care should be taken to set this against the rest of the dream.

Violet, and all its subtle variations, is fairly unusual for dreams. It is generally connected with one's inner self, unless, of course, it is a rather factual dream where you are picking a bunch of violets. Even so, dreams such as these can be interpreted on more levels than one. To dream of purple robes may mean aspirations of power or success, while to dream of amethysts denotes a healing situation. Generally, violet is a color connected with spirituality and one's inner life.

Brown in dreams gives a rather dull, negative quality. It can suggest all the earthly qualities of rocks, soil, mud—together with the possibilities of being bogged down, stuck in a rut, or just plodding along—or even a time of aridity, depending on the shade in question. All-brown dreams are fairly uncommon and would perhaps reveal that the dreamer is browned-off with life or going through a dull period.

All-**Gray** dreams emphasize similar possibilities to all-brown dreams and indicate a very dreary mental outlook. In smaller quantities, however, both colors have their place in normally colored dreams.

Black in dreams does not necessarily mean something dire. A black cat crossing one's path points to some good luck coming. A black human figure can represent the unconscious or sexual side of ourselves. Black animals, depending on the nature of the creature, can be beautiful or menacing depending on the "feel" of the dream, Black in dreams should be set against the other aspects and interpreted accordingly.

White in dreams is not usually seen exclusively, unless it is a snow scene. If you recall such a dream setting it could imply some "freezing" of the emotions, and if everything is completely iced up, then you have a bit of a problem! Try melting some of that snow and ice so that little rivers and green fields can appear!

The most rewarding dreams are, of course, those in several colors. One main color in an otherwise monochrome dream usually pinpoints a significant aspect, but a whole range of color suggests balance and harmony. Taken along with a generally positive content, this is the most enjoyable kind of dream to have but, alas, all too rare for most people.

MEDITATION

Meditation is a somewhat different activity to that of dreaming, although there are similarities. The former is usually controlled, the latter only occasionally. While meditating, one can call up a particular color, either for general contemplation or for a particular purpose, such as healing. Then there are the colors that float through one's mind or are associated with the object of meditation. Most meditation teachers instruct students to ignore these passing diversions, but it might be worthwhile to briefly note them in passing and later check on their specific meanings, although undue importance should not be attached to them.

A meditation on a specific color is often a useful exercise. The color can generally be visualized either as filling the immediate surroundings, as a cloud in front of one's eyes, or embodied in something symbolic such as a rose, a cup, a pool, a tree, and so on. Care should be taken to remember that the object chosen for the color in question has its own symbolic associations, and if you just wish to contemplate pure color, then choose a very simple geometrical shape. Color cards are a useful prop for this kind of meditation, because you can gaze at a particular color for some moments and fix it in your mind's eye. Then visualize it mentally and see what comes.

Another interesting exercise is to take a color card, without looking to see what color it is, and place it face down on a table. Then "tune in" to it and see what comes. This exercise, like any other ESP test, is best done in a small group or with another person. The results can be very illuminating and can give you much symbolic imagery to play with afterward. You may not perceive the actual color of the card, but you will probably get some sort of sensation with it as described in the earlier section on sightless vision.

A worthwhile area of experimentation is that of mind games. These are not quite meditation in the usual meaning of the word, but they certainly overlap in some areas. A mind game is to some extent a "talk-through" meditation; in another sense it stretches the mind and exercises quite a few dormant faculties. "Path-working" is another term used for this type of activity, but whatever you call it the results can be very beneficial.

You may like to try such a game, incorporating color visualization as well as using your imagination for the other senses of touch, smell, and hearing. With the correct formula and a good leader, a group of people can return form such an excursion both refreshed and relaxed. It isn't hypnosis and you are totally in command of your own version of the game. But it is important for the leader to take it fairly slowly, giving people the chance to arrange their inner scenery. A typical example would be as follows. I call it "Eternity."

The leader first suggests that everyone seat themselves in a comfortable and relaxed position, with feet firmly on the ground and hands gently resting on the knees. A few deep breaths and/or a body consciousness exercise will put the participants in the right frame of mind, turning them away from all thoughts of mundane problems. The body consciousness exercise consists of relaxing each part of the body in turn, commencing with the feet and going on up to the top of the head. This can be combined with closing the aura by visualizing a blue or white light encircling the body, topped with a protective symbol such as a cross (or whatever you prefer). This exercise leaves everyone feeling comfortably relaxed and yet protected, with their train of everyday thoughts broken and dispersed. After a little practice this exercise takes only a few minutes or so, and then the leader can suggest the following exercise.

You are walking along the beach on a beautiful sunny day. The sky is an intense blue with a few fluffy white clouds floating around; the sea is sparkling. You can smell the saltiness in the air and feel the crunchiness of the yellow sand beneath your bare feet; hear the swish of the small wavelets as they ebb and flow; feel the golden warmth of the sunshine. In the distance you can see white cliffs topped with green grass. As you walk along you feel a little breeze brushing your face. After a while you come to a pathway leading away from the beach and up toward the top of the cliff. It is rocky but not too steep, and as you climb upward you pass clumps of pink sea-thrift and brilliant scarlet poppies growing among the chalky rocks. The path finally leads you to the top of the cliff. You are above the sea now, surrounded by lush, green grass, daisies and poppies, and other flowers. You sit down gratefully, relax, and gaze out to the sea. The scintillating stillness of the ocean, reflecting gold and silver lights, and the calm blue of the sky combine to give you a sense of eternity, timelessness, and utter security. You think on this idea for a little while (3–5 minutes) as you enjoy the colors and sensations around you. After this short rest, rise and return to the rocky path that leads to the beach, all the while continuing to sense the qualities of air, earth, water, and fire and seeing the colors of your surroundings. Once back on the beach, take one last look at the ocean and then let the scene fade from your mind. You are now back in your chair, feeling refreshed and relaxed.

Make sure that you are properly "earthed" by stretching and wriggling about a bit and by imagining that your aura is still enclosing you. It wouldn't do to remain on Cloud Nine—you might not notice where you were going on the way home or you might end up feeling rather disassociated.

This sort of exercise makes a very pleasant end to an evening of discussion, healing, or listening to music. It enlarges your color visualization capabilities and makes you more aware of a lot of things you take for granted. An enterprising leader can modify the exercise by introducing additional touches such as some little sailing ships with colored sails or beach huts in brilliant colors; or the leader can extend the walk to take in a rather more complicated scenario. You can stop to bathe in the sea, if you wish, or even take a swim. For those people who say "I can't stand heights" or "I'm frightened of water," the leader must give encouragement and help by explaining that they have complete control over their "picture" and can modify it or shut it off, whenever they like. The leader should stress that this type of exercise offers a wonderful opportunity to overcome such hang-ups and that by mentally approaching whatever it is that is frightening the sufferer can gradually gain control over it. This sort of exercise is sometimes used in aversion therapy, although maybe not with such pleasant spin-offs as a nice day at the seaside.

Yet another exercise can enhance your color awareness, besides giving you some insights into your own subconscious. This I call "The Treasure Cave."

This time, after the usual relaxation procedure, we find ourselves standing outside a cave (those frightened of caves can have a torch or take a gnome with them for company, if they like). It is an attractive cave, with little green ferns growing around its mouth and a silver stream trickling down beside it. You enter the cave, which has a faint luminosity of its own so that you can see your way. It is cool inside, and the path is slightly sandy. The sides of the tunnel are smooth and now and again you can see the same little green ferns that were growing outside. You walk along the tunnel, which is gradually descending, lower and lower. (Give a little time here for everyone to make their descent.) Eventually, the tunnel widens and you are standing in a vast cave with many twinkling points of light, illuminating the cavern sufficiently to reveal, in front of you, a still, small pool of clear water. You go toward the pool and sit down beside it, gazing into it. It is not very deep and has a sandy bottom. Lying on the bottom are many colored precious stones—amethyst, ruby, pearl, sapphire, emerald, opal, diamond, topaz—together with such semiprecious substances as amber and coral. (You can make this as simple or as complicated as you like.) You are allowed to take one of these stones. You put your hand into the water (try to feel its wetness and coolness) and take out the stone of your choice. Let us say it is a sapphire. It is a fairly large stone, the size of a walnut. You gaze into its blue depths, and it is as if looking into a blue grotto. There is the same sense of timelessness and endurance as we had at the sea, plus the stability and comfort of the earth. You take your stone with you as you rise from beside the pool and retrace your steps back along the tunnel, again reliving the sensation of coolness, smooth walls, sandy floor. You emerge from the cave mouth into soft, warm sunshine to see your chair just outside the cave. Sit in it and come back gently to the present, using the same techniques as before for earthing yourself.

You have brought a gift back with you this time—your sapphire. Now, you can look up any good book of symbology (see Further Reading) and find out for yourself the meaning of a sapphire. But in case you haven't such a reference book at hand, here are a few brief notes on the meanings of such jewels.

Amethyst—Humility, peace of mind, sobriety; the stone of healing; bringer of dreams and visions; protection against over enthusiasm.

Amber—Congealed light; courage; gives magic power and protection; sacred to Apollo and regarded as Freya's tears.

Coral—Sea-tree of the Mother Goddess; longevity, fertility of the waters, ideas, aspiration.

Diamond—Light, life, the sun, constancy, innocence, eternity, incorruptibility, durability, eternity of spirit.

Emerald—Immortality, hope, youth; spring, growth of spiritual awareness, harmony with life.

Opal—Faithfulness, religious intensity, prayers, psychic powers; protection against anger, purification.

Pearl—Chastity, purity, the moon, feminine principle, value, beauty that arises from the trials of life.

Ruby—Dignity, power, love, passion, beauty, longevity, invulnerability, sympathy, feeling for others.

Sapphire—Truth, chastity, spirituality, contemplation and devotion, protection from evil, heavenly attributes.

Topaz—Divine goodness, fidelity, friendship, love, sagacity, the sun.

This list should give you some food for thought. Why did you choose such a stone? Was it the color that attracted you or some other association? Combined with the meanings in the above list and with the color meanings given earlier, you should be able to compile yourself quite a useful little dossier about why you like a particular color, thus gaining some insight into your inner self. Jewels traditionally symbolize spiritual truths, and jewels from a cave refer to the intuitive knowledge hidden in the unconscious.

You may wonder what such exercises have to do with healing, but rest assured, anything that relaxes the body, stimulates the mind, and refreshes the spirit is healing. Whatever our state of health, all of us can do with a little healing of one sort or another at times—the stresses of everyday modern life, with its vast range of choices and many complications, often make us tense and anxious without knowing it. A little break now and then reminds us of our priorities. You may like to try another exercise. I call this "Belonging."

Begin with the usual relaxation procedure, and then imagine you are standing on a beautiful sandy beach in the early hours of the morning, just before the sun is up. All is quiet except for the gentle ripple of the waves on the shore. You can see the crescent moon and many stars high in the sky. As you gaze toward the horizon, the first faint light of dawn is appearing, a pale pink flush of color, and the deep blue of the night sky above you becomes paler—a translucent eggshell blue. Slowly the stars begin to disappear as the dawn light creeps upward. All, that is, except one star, which is the most brilliant. It gives out great flashes of color—red, green, blue, and gold—like a diamond. You contemplate it, knowing that you and it are eternally linked, that you are made of the same star-stuff forged eons ago and trillions of light years away. You are composed of the same material as that great star, which is now sending huge shafts of light down to you; both of you were created in the first great dawn when the universe began.

This star, this cosmic "relative," has a message for you. It sends out one final great amethyst flash of light as the sky lightens. This amethyst light reaches down to where you are standing, and for a moment you and the star are indissolubly linked. Experience the feeling of belonging in the universe, of being part of it, of knowing you are a child of the stars and that you have a right to be here as much as that vast sun. You are at one with it as a member of the universe. Thank the star for its message and, as it finally winks out, turn to look at the sun rising over the horizon. Salute it, as a fellow being, then let the scene fade from your mind and return to your present environment, making sure your aura is "closed" and you are properly earthed.

The "message" this great star sends you may not be an obvious one. It may leave you with an enhanced experience of cosmic consciousness, or something may surface later in your mind or in a dream. You could try other colors in this exercise and see if you get different results.

Here I suggest a final exercise, one in which you can assess how much knowledge you have acquired about color so far and whether you can use this knowledge in a positive way. It is called "The Castle."

Commence with the usual relaxation procedure. Them imagine you are walking on a little path across a meadow toward a white castle in the distance. The day is warm and sunny, the meadow is lush and green, full of wildflowers, chirping crickets, and humming bees. There is a peaceful and serene atmosphere. The path is leading you up to the castle, which is fairly large. It has six doorways and over each hangs a beautiful silk flag, each a different color—scarlet, yellow, soft green, blue, indigo, and violet. Choose one of the doorways and enter the castle. You go up six short steps and enter a hall. This hall is completely colored in whatever color flag was hanging over the door you chose—floor, walls, furniture, and even the light filtering through leaded panes is colored. You feel completely immersed in this color, almost as if you are breathing it in. Try to feel its qualities, its warmth or coolness, its stimulation or tranquility. Feel that the very air around you is colored. Take what you need from it. Presently, pass through the hall to a door at the far end. Climb another short flight of stairs and this time you enter a hall of pure crystal which reflects back to you many scintillating colors. Here is the heart of your castle. Now take whatever you feel was the best in your color and place it, in the form of a symbol, on a table in the center of the hall. The symbol can take any form: a fruit, a flower, an abstract design. Choose it to portray the qualities of your color choice. This is your gift to your castle. It lies there secure for you whenever you wish to return. Return through the castle and meadow and finish as before.

A castle represents our inner security and that which is difficult to attain; it usually holds some treasure. You can use such an exercise to go through the whole color spectrum. This exercise will help your color visualization immensely and will fix in your mind the qualities associated with the different colors. It may also give you a pleasant feeling of relaxation and well-being if you are in a mood you would like to change. If you feel your mind needs to be stimulated, choose the red of yellow flags; if you need calming, try the blue or green; if you really need to lift your consciousness, try the indigo and violet.

What actually comes forth after such mind games and the simple meditation techniques described in this chapter is subject to your own personal interpretation, and it is important not to ask someone else to do this for you unless you are really stuck for an answer. The value of the exercise will be lost otherwise. Considering a particular color may bring scenes and symbols to your mind of a personal nature. Blue, for instance, may bring memories and associations that may surprise you with their depth. On the other hand, such associations may surprise you with their triviality. But deep or shallow, they are all part of you and worthy of attention. This kind of meditation is fairly low-key, but even so it can provide valuable insights into one's inner life.

5 COLOR IN OUR HEALING

Color healing of one type or another has been popular from very early days when color was first used for symbolic reasons. The ancient Egyptians, Babylonians, and Assyrians practiced therapeutic sunbathing, and a highly developed sun and airbathing cult existed in ancient Greece and Rome. The old Germanic races likewise regarded the healing power of sunlight very highly and worshiped the rising sun. The Incas of South America also practiced a sun cult called heliotherapy.[1] It is obvious that in these long ago times people were as well aware of the healing value of sunlight as we are today. This may seem to have no direct connection with actual color healing until we remember that sunlight can be split into the colors of the spectrum and thus contains all of these within itself.

The decision to use individual colors in the form of light rays for specific healing problems must have originated along with the use of plants, flowers, pigments, and so forth of a color corresponding to the disease in question; for example, red flowers, among others, were used to treat a blood condition.As this aspect of healing developed, someone along the way had the idea that colored light might have a similarly efficacious effect.

In the first century A.D. Aurelius Cornelius Celsus wrote a number of books on medicine which included various colored ointments and plasters in black, green, and white. Claudius Galen, Greek physician to Marcus Aurelius (a most celebrated medical writer), mentions color in his treatises. Avicenna (980–1037), an Arabian philosopher and physician and author of the book *Canon of Medicine*, considered color most important in diagnosis, relating it to the human temperament and the physical state of the body. He maintained, for instance, that to gaze at something red if one were bleeding would make matters worse. Like Celsus, Avicenna used colored flowers in his remedies, matching them by color to the ailments in question.

Then along came a German–Swiss physician and chemist, Theothrastus Bombastus von Hohenheim, who assumed the name of Paracelsus. His theories were much advanced for his time, but he didn't have a very good opinion of Galen and Avicenna and publicly burned their books. Even so, color was included among the many remedies he used, along with music, herbs, diet, bleeding and purging, and so on.

Since then there have been many practitioners of color healing of varying degrees of credibility. One of the most outstanding was Edwin D. Babbitt, who was enthusiastically acclaimed by many people but attacked by the medical profession. His book, *The Principles of Light and Color* (1878), created quite a sensation in the field of color healing. He claimed cures of various ailments by the treatment of sunlight passed through panes of colored glass, and he invented and sold such aids to color healing as "Chromo-Disks," "Chromo-flasks," a "Thermolume" cabinet for color therapy treatment, and a type of stained glass window that could also be used for color healing purposes. He set up a chain of correspondences between colors and the elements and minerals. Babbitt was not quite the first in his field, but he was certainly one of the most spectacular exponents of color healing.

Babbitt considered blue and violet to have soothing qualities, and therefore regarded them as useful for all inflammatory and nervous conditions, while white and blue were regarded as good for sciatica and rheumatism. (You will see later in the chapter that this does not tie in with much present-day thinking.) Along with many others, Babbitt considered red to have a potent effect upon the blood and to be very helpful in cases of paralysis, while yellow and orange stimulated the nerves. Various arrangements of these colors were used for more complex conditions. His basic principles, however, are still used today by many color therapy practitioners, some of whom have developed their own versions of his original work.

Naturally, the subject remains a matter of controversy, and although Babbitt's chromotherapeutic devices and prescriptions are not legally allowed in the United States, his country of origin, in Britian there is a fairly wide choice of color therapists who use and sell his aids to color therapy.

Perhaps a few words on cosmic rays would be appropriate at this point. Many healers talk about working with these "rays," which may seem puzzling to the uninitiated. These rays are, of course, those of the light spectrum—the colors of the rainbow. Each ray is regarded as having certain attributes and on the whole these attributes tie in fairly well with color meanings already outlined. Many healers add to the seven spectrum rays the colors brown, gray, black, and white, sometimes adding an extra shade or two of any one color. In order to keep matters simple, however, we shall identify only eleven of the rays.

When a healer works with a certain color ray, then he or she intends to utilize all the known positive characteristics of that particular ray. Extra ammunition—in the form of similarly colored plants, flowers, vegetables, and fruit, and color-charged water, colored lamps, and even colored clothes—is brought in to reinforce the positive characteristics of the ray. Most deities are associated with one or more of the color rays, and this is where those who engage in ritual of any kind find it important to correlate in color all the impediments used in the ritual. For others, strong visualization of the color required will be sufficient, and while one does not think each time, "red—that's warmth, life, energy, and so on," obviously the person using the rays must have some basic idea of what they represent. To sum up, talk of working with cosmic rays is really just a rather fancy way of saying you are working with certain color principles. Let us begin with the basics.

Red includes every shade and tint from pink to maroon. It is regarded as the ray of will and power, life, vitality, and energy. It is also symbolic of blood, battles, and war, and red ray qualities can be found in the symbolism of religious and spiritual movements, signifying the fight against evil. Much talk is made of people being "on a certain ray." If you feel you are on a red ray, then you're the pioneering, leader type of person (or would like to be). Red is regarded by some healers as a powerful healing agent in diseases of the blood and circulation, general debility, and depression; it also inspires heroism and courage.

Orange is the ray associated with energy. It has some modified characteristics of the red ray, bringing thought (yellow) to action (red). It therefore brings in qualities of discipline and control to the wilder attributes of red and in some ways has a more practical flavor to it. This color, however, should be used carefully—not many people can carry it off well. Nervy people should avoid it. It is thought to be helpful for chest conditions, problems of the spleen and kidneys, and for digestive ailments.

Yellow is the ray of intellect, mental creativity, and a liking for mental employment and activity as opposed to the physical. It is thought to have a stimulating effect on the nerves and is related to the great glandular center at the solar plexus. Yellow ray people are usually very quick thinkers. At its highest level it is the ray of wisdom, although, unfortunately, it does have some rather dismal connotations. In the main it is a very stimulating ray. It has a powerful effect on the nervous system and is considered suitable for a room where mental pursuits are undertaken. Some healers use this ray for diseases of the skin and nerves.

Green is the ray of balance, harmony and sympathy, adaptability, and diplomacy. Used wisely, it should ideally sort out different levels of a situation so that a suitable compromise is reached. It can be a good tonic for tired nerves, and its changeable quality also helps prevent stagnation. There is, however, the danger that green ray people may find themselves sitting on both sides of the fence at once! Green is a mixture of blue-yellow (love-wisdom), and it is said to influence the heart center, healing and soothing emotional disorders and nervous headaches. It is, to a great extent, the color of our planet, and gazing at green fields, trees, and plants has a very soothing effect. Even so, for the highly nervous it may not have such a beneficial result, as in the case of someone who was unhappy living in the country and who really required a more stimulating environment. Sometimes the force of nature can be overwhelming to people who are not in a good state of balance, and as such, although it is a ray of inexhaustible energy, it must be used with care.

Blue is usually regarded as the "love" ray on its highest plane. It symbolizes harmony, truth, and serenity and helps raise the consciousness to a spiritual level. It soothes and calms the mind, but it can be rather cool. Thus, blue can be used for cleansing, for fighting feverish conditions, bleeding, and nervous irritations. All the characteristics of blue come together in this ray, which is only superseded by its higher counterpart, indigo, the ray of spirituality, devotion, intuition, and dedication. Indigo holds a hint of mystery and can at times be cold and dispassionate, but a true indigo, like the evening sky, suggests inner light of a quality to offset cooler attributes. It is astringent, purifying, and said to influence the organs of sight, hearing, and smell and thus is used for diseases of the eye, ear, and nose.

Amethyst is the ray connected with ceremony, ritual, and magic but also that of spiritual and mental equilibrium. It is a useful ray for tranquilizing a troubled situation. This ray influences the highest in humans and can be spiritually healing and purifying, aiding sleep and the development of psychic abilities. Those rare folk on a true amethyst ray are the peacemakers in the world.

Purple and **Violet** follow, with more of red (will and power) accompanying the qualities of spirituality and calmness, so it is not surprising that they are used so much for ritual, both secular and religious. On its lower levels purple and violet can indicate pride and pomposity, but on the violet end it is considered equivalent to the highest and most evolved state of consciousness. No wonder, as you will see later, it helps "repel nasty spirits"! Violet is used by some for the treatment of mental and nervous problems, neuralgia, rheumatism, and epilepsy.

Brown is similar to green in that it is a ray of balance, but it has to be used with discretion. The term "brown study" aptly describes its qualities of concentration and acquisition of knowledge. It can be rather heavy, but small quantities are essential to "earth" a situation or personality that has become rather out of hand.

Gray, at its highest silvery hue, is the ray of peace; darker shades indicated persistence and spiritual struggle. There are some people who seem to be silver ray people—if of the silvery hue, there seems something mercurial, light, and elusive about them; on the darker level they are just as difficult to get through to but of a denser vibration.

Black, while obviously not used in orthodox healing, still has a place among the other rays. Its purpose is to absorb and store away secretly—much as the color black absorbs all other colors, giving none out. Its restrictive and protective qualities are useful for those who wish to keep their mysteries hidden from the gaze of the uninitiated. Perhaps if you are on this ray you are an aspiring magician of a very secret order!

The above is, of course, a very simplified list of the meanings attributed to the color rays. It does not not mean that because you like a certain color, you are "on" that ray. It takes honest self-examination, and maybe an even more honest friend, before one can really be considered on a certain ray. In fact, most of us are a mixture of rays, in this sense, with perhaps one more predominant than the others. Suggestions for those who wish to study the subject more in depth are given at the end of the chapter.

This discussion should give you some idea of how cosmic rays are used. For healing, these rays can be applied for their qualities on all levels—mental, physical, and spiritual.

Practical Aids

One of the most well-known color therapists in Britain is Theo Gimbel who runs the Hygeia Clinic in Gloucester and who has published a number of books on the subject of color healing. Gimbel's father, Max Gümbel-Seiling, worked with Rudolf Steiner between 1912 and

1925. They evolved a system of colors for stage lighting and practical use whereby appropriate colors can be made to suggest certain atmospheres; for example, a rainbow for spirituality; black and gray for a somber or macabre situation; red for joyful activity; blue for sympathy, devotion, and so on. White suggests angels and brides, while black is reminiscent of a priest, a judge, or the devil. Gray reminds us of ghosts, dusk and dawn, and all in-between states; violet, magic and mystical states; brown, down to earth and matter-of-fact things. The Anthroposophical Society, of which Rudolph Steiner was the founder, has done an immense amount of work on various types of color therapy, particularly in the field of artistic expression. Gimbel has obviously been much influenced by the society's work, and that of Babbitt to some extent, but he has clearly expanded on both these methods and evolved a comprehensive system of his own. He maintains, for instance, that children up to the age of three or so see colors in their complementaries—if looking at green the child will see magenta. He believes, therefore, that pregnant women should wear white, orange, or red as these colors do not interfere with the natural (reversed) perception of the embryo. As an embryo, accordingly, the only color we experience is a deep blue. This ties in somewhat with Dr. Bucke's theories of the evolution of the color sence. It might also explain why blue is such a significant color inasmuch as one wishes to "sink into it" if one is feeling stressed; it might be a desire to return to the womb.

Gimbel also assigns various colors to different areas of the spine, giving corresponding link-ups with music and astrology. He considers the connection between the spine and the sound of the whole human skeleton to be most significant. Among the aids to therapy he uses are 16 different filters that form part of the treatment in his color therapy room, which is generally bathed in a blue light filtered through variously shaped apertures onto whichever part of the body needs healing. Gimbel's books give clear instructions for proceeding with color therapy on a purely mental basis, but it would undoubtedly prove more valuable to undergo a training period at his clinic. This system of color filters for chromotherapy is quite popular, and most healers either use a lamp or projector into which the filters can be inserted or ask the patient to sit in a Dr. Babbitt-type "Thermolume" cabinet and be bathed in color from various screens fixed at the front of it.

Another widely used method for color therapy is one of wrapping a color filter around a glass of water and placing it in the sunlight for an hour or so. The patient then drinks the water or uses it to bathe any afflicted areas. This is one of the methods favored by the College of Psychotherapeutics, White Lodge, Spalding, Kent, where it is also possible to stay for the purposes of treatment and/or study.

A variation on the above methods is used at the Château de Relaxarium at Mazerolles-du-Razes in France, where patients can lie and sunbathe comfortably under color filter screens. These treatments are coordinated with yoga and other therapeutic exercises in peaceful country surroundings.

A system combining color therapy and yoga is outlined by Annie Wilson and Lilla Bek in their book *What Color Are You?*[2] The authors work on the chakric centers of the body through various yoga exercises. Detailed instructions and photographs outline this system of therapy. I strongly feel, however, that yoga needs to be personally taught, otherwise one may adopt an incorrect position that may be difficult to eradicate and that may do more harm than good.

CHAKRIC HEALING

Many color healers work on the chakric points. The chakras are places in the auric body where energy is centralized, as it were. Usually regarded as seven in number, they are seen clairvoyantly as whirling vortices of light. If well balanced and working properly, them it's "all systems go," but if not, it is assumed that a rebalancing treatment is neccessary. The chakras tend to influence the part of the physical body in which they are situated, and their colors and attributes correspond to the rainbow spectrum, as follows, so it is easy enough to remember them.

LOCATION	COLOR	ATTRIBUTE
Crown of head/pituitary	Violet	Spirituality/philosophy
Forehead (third eye)/pineal	Blue	Clairvoyance
Throat-Thyroid	Turquoise	Intelligence/clairaudience
Heart	Green	Understanding/compassion
Stomach/solarplexus	Yellow	Feeling
Adrenals/side kidneys	Orange	Feeling/sensation
Sacral/base of spine	Red	Sexual energy/procreation

Healing to the chakra in question is usually given in the form of color replenishment. The chakras are, however, usually in a very delicate state of balance, and inexperienced healers should not attempt to interfere with them or they could make matters worse. Many healers combine yoga and massage with chakric color therapy.

In her excellent book *Color Healing,* Mary Anderson recommends color breathing, which she considers as important as the drinking of color-charged water. One is shown, by means of instructions in the book, how to breathe in the required color. Again, the chakras are an important link with the color therapy, but the author does advise that a color therapist be consulted. Generally, the treatments follow the line of color correspondences, as when red fruit and vegetables are combined with red-charged water for conditions such as anemia, with further treatment of red light applied to the soles of the feet and to the "red" chakras at the base of the spine. Many other illustrations are given for treatment along the lines described.

The author briefly describes a system of gem therapy practiced in India. The gems are set in a rotating disc in such a way that their rays will fall on a patient's photograph. This method does not fall into the usual color correspondence system, apart from the ruby, which is considered to resonate to the red cosmic ray and the sun and is therefore used for treating heart diseases, anemia, and similar complaints. Dr. Bhattacharyya, the exponent of this particular system, considers pearl (the moon) to reflect the orange cosmic ray; coral (Mars), the yellow cosmic ray; and so on. He has two interesting big guns he brings in, however—the onyx, which is said to carry the ultraviolet frequency, and the cat's eye, which carries the infra red frequency.

Anderson outlines another system of working with colors—numbers and music, with correspondences in fruit and vegetables depending on the particular cosmic ray used.

Perfume can also be combined with color and music for healing purposes, and such a method is described in Roland Hunt's *Fragrant and Radiant Healing Symphony*.[4] Again, the author works with cosmic rays and their correspondences in perfume, music, and colored lamps.

Then there is a method of healing by crystals, which can be charged with either pure white light or whatever color is required. This is available from the Crystal Healing Centre[5] at Sherborne, Dorset, and this type of healing is used to correct chakric imbalances and is frequently combined with yoga, massage, and various other alternative remedies. In this instance, crystals may afford some measure of amplification for healing energies.

It is possible to try a few experiments for yourself with colored lights to see how they affect your mood and general well-being. Try red or orange, and to a lesser extent yellow, to raise body temperature and to cheer yourself up or stimulate your mind. You will probably find that short time in such drastic lighting is quite enough. Bright green or blue light will slow the heartbeat and lower body temperature, but it may not be advisable to switch from one to the other too suddenly. Many shops provide an opportunity to experience first hand such sudden changes of "atmosphere," so it is not at all necessary to put oneself to the expense of buying specially colored lamps when these sensations can be tried for free!

"Mind Power" Color Healing

From these rather practical aids to color therapy we come to the healers who use color in a more subjective sense—that of visualizing and sending color either in direct or absent healing. Many healers use this method and have their own interpretations of color by which they work. However, I am only going to describe one such method in detail here—the method used by the Atlanteans.

The Atlanteans is a philosophical organization with interest in all

New Age subjects including meditation, self-awareness, ESP, the Nature Kingdoms, and, of course, Atlantis. One of its primary functions is that of healing—self-healing as well as healing of other people. Before we dip too deeply into their healing methods, we shall consider a few other opinions. We have seen how in the past color awareness has developed, particularly in regard to healing, and we can see how the various correspondences have built up between ailments and the plants, fruits, and so on used to cure them. This still applies in color healing by mind power, although each healer tends to make an individual interpretation.

Most healers tend to agree that blue is a healing, cleansing, and calming color. White also is often used for general healing. This is the point where healers tend to part company, for use of colors beyond these two is widely individual. As an Atlantean healer, I might be horrified at the idea of sending red to anyone except for a specific purpose(described later). But some healers find it very useful for treating depression, anemia, and similar conditions. Yellow is a fairly controversial color (I am not here equating it with the sun or "golden light"), but, according to one school of thought, it stimulates mental powers and circulates energy. Green, a color to be used with some caution as it can be rather depressive, is suggested as good for the expectant mothers,[6] and it may well be, as used by this particular school of thought. It only goes to show how widely divergent are the opinions of color therapists. Some suggestions are rather simplistic, such as purple (a color with religious connotations) repelling nasty spirits. As a first line of defense, however, it is very useful. Many healers recommend surrounding a patient with light which, of course, includes all colors. This is an excellent suggestion, but for those who wish to be a little more specific, a course of color healing would be the best way of getting off on the right foot. Color healing can be quite complex, and if you start off with a hit-and-miss attitude, you probably won't do much harm, but you won't do much good either. It is far better to get some initial practical training first hand. As you become more experienced you can begin to develop your own style. Most healers agree, however, that red and green must be used very carefully; blue and turquoise are about the most helpful for relaxing the body and cleansing; yellow and orange, while revitalizing, have to be used sparingly.

The Atlanteans take the view that for specific healing cases it is necessary to work with at least one or two other persons and that in the beginning at least one of the group should have had some personal tuition. However good correspondence courses are, there is nothing like being shown how to do something and being able to ask questions and compare notes. Unfortunately, there are many people who would love to do this and who have a great desire to help in the world, but who are unable, for reasons of location, work, or domestic difficulties, to join a group or take part in residential courses. The Atlanteans have produced a course for such people[7] which, while it does not include the detailed instruction given to healers in a group, is sufficiently structured so as to give a frame of reference from which to begin. Six simple lessons give basic instruction in care of the aura, concentration, meditation, visualization, and techniques of prayer and absent healing, designed in a way to protect the student and to concentrate the healing powers not only on others but on oneself.

It might appear from this course that too great an emphasis is placed on protection of healer and patient, and many people ask, "What is there to be afraid of?" and "If healing is sent with love, what can cause harm?"—all very nice sentiments but a little unrealistic. The best of intentions does not guarantee you immunity from either physical or mental "invaders," and it is only sensible to take reasonable precautions. Very few of us are adepts, able to walk through the world and, by the power of our thoughts, pass unharmed through all kinds of dangers. Would you wander around a slum area, known for its muggings and violence, without some form of defense unless you had to? Do you leave your front door or car unlocked? Love alone won't keep burglars at bay, you have to take precautions on all levels—lock the door on the physical level; put a strong thought, prayer, or whatever for the protection of the property on a mental level, and finally, if you wish, leave a thought of love for whoever is so out of balance with themselves as to want to injure someone else's property, thus completing the three levels of physical, mental, and spiritual. Of course, we all take chances, hoping it won't happen to us. I for one certainly do not always remember, after locking the door, either of the other two precautions! (For those who wish to investigate these ideas in greater depth I suggest reading Murry Hope's book *Practical Techniques of Psychic Self Defense* [see Further Reading]. Hope is one of the founding members of the Atlanteans and as such has these techniques at her fingertips.[8])

With healing, it is very important that you are protected on all three levels, and it is wiser not to take chances. In my early days of healing, I heard a number of cases where well-meaning inexperienced healers had tried to help someone by "drawing off" a malignant illness. In one instance, at least, the patient recovered and the healer got the disease instead. One psychic magazine regularly relates anxious queries about what can be done to throw off a condition picked up from a patient. In one issue[9] a reader states that after practicing healing on a friend, "I had great difficulty in breathing and realized that the person healed had suffered from a chest complaint." If the healer is experienced, this can probably be thrown off without too much difficulty; but if the healer is inexperienced, then it may prove much more difficult. Isn't it easier to take precautions to begin with? These are extreme cases, of course, but it can happen.

There is no fear motivation behind the teaching of protective measures in Atlantean healing, only sensible precautions. Sometimes healers can pass things on to patients that the patients may not want, and although most people unconsciously reject any unwanted transmissions of any nature, an ailing or seriously ill person would not have a strong defense mechanism and might be unable to resist.

ATLANTEAN HEALING TECHNIQUE

The most basic level on which to prepare yourself for healing is, naturally, the physical one. To be in in a comfortable position, relaxed but alert, not hungry but not having just eaten a heavy meal, will set the scene for perhaps the most important aspect of Atlantean healing—the control of the aura. The course describes in some detail the functions of the aura and how to keep it good health.

To start with, one undertakes a body consciousness exercise beginning at the feet and slowly upward, becoming aware of and relaxing each part of the body in turn, until the top of the head is reached. If your mind happens to wander during this exercise, then you will have to start again from the feet. After this has been successfully completed, you can do the exercise again, this time drawing up around yourself blue or white light until you are completely cocooned in it. If you find this difficult, you can imagine stepping into a blue plastic bag, drawing it up around yourself, and sealing it at the top with a cross or ankh or whatever symbol you would normally use for protection. It is extremely important, however, that you be as relaxed as possible, and if you complete the body consciousness exercise correctly, you should be feeling very relaxed. You can also take a few deep breaths as well. This technique is used for patients as well as healers working on their own, as a patient receiving direct healing who is in an unrelaxed state is not likely to receive much benefit from healing.

Of course, the aura is an emanation from the spirit and as such is always radiating from the body, but the above exercise will reinforce and strengthen it. Be aware that your mind can control it. You can try a few auric color changes and ask a fellow healer what color they see. You can blow your aura out or completely withdraw it so that it cannot be seen, but whatever you do, don't forget it! Always do your healing through the filter of your aura—you can imagine it as a very fine mesh that only lets through the highest cosmic energies. If you suspect it has been damaged, either do the body consciousness exercise on yourself, strongly visualizing that the affected part is being repaired, or get another healer to do so. Even a small cut causes the aura to break, and it should be repaired immediately. You can do this for yourself by drawing on the cosmic energies, imagining them coming down through your aura and through the top of your head and down and out through your fingertips. Hold your hands for a couple of minutes (it seems quite a long time) over the site of the injury and imagine the energy repairing the tear in the aura, a bit like darning a sock. Perhaps the following example will give you some idea of how it works.

A friend of mine, who besides being an Atlantean healer has also been a nurse, was talking one day (during a tea break, of course) to the Works Sister at her place of employment. They had previously discussed healing and my friend had been explaining that Atlantean healing mostly means work on the aura. "Is the aura that light I can see around everyone," suddenly asked Sister, "and why does it have a break in it if someone hurts themselves?" She said she had seen this "light" around people for many years but did not know what it meant. My friend explained, and mentioned healing the aura, as described above. "Oh, just a minute then," said the Sister, popping out of the room. She came back with a cut on her finger that was bleeding. "Can you heal that?" she asked. My friend began visualizing energy streaming from her hands. She held them above the cut finger, sealing off the small cut in the aura. "I can see a blue light coming from your hands," said Sister, "the bleeding has stopped too." Unfortunately, this woman became rather frightened about her ability to see the aura and thereafter tended to avoid the subject. Perhaps one day she will be able to look at the whole subject in an objective manner.

This is a fairly simple illustration of how a break in the aura can be sealed—and also how someone can see the aura without actually knowing it. For cases of extreme shock and general injury, as compared with minor problems, one would need to be able to visualize the whole of the aura, realign it with the body, and seal it carefully. This would best be done by an experienced healer or group of healers. This technique is, however, very useful for lesser bumps, bruises, and burns. Speaking from experience, it can be very effective, often preventing a bruise or burn if caught in time. Blue or white light can be used, although some healers use a colorless ray. It all depends how you feel about a particular case.

White covers a broad area in Atlantean healing. It can be used to recharge and seal the aura, for yourself or someone else. In fact, most simple physical problems can be dealt with by white or blue. Sometimes there is a necessity for a soothing, gentle color for relief of pain and tension. Here we use coral and pink with its suggestion of warmth and comfort. Sometimes it takes a bit of practice to achieve this color, whereas red is easier to visualize, but you certainly wouldn't use that for soothing. Red, in fact, is rarely used in Atlantean healing, and is instead reserved for certain ulcerous conditions that need drying up. It is never used for any type of mental healing.

Lilac is occasionally used, but it is rather "heavy" and needs a good build-up of power to achieve any potency. It is, therefore, best left to experienced healers. Its function is to replenish and rebuild.

Green, as mentioned before, is only used sparingly. It can be used to calm the overactive or even violent person, but it is not considered suitable for people suffering from nervous tension or cases of depression, as it may create even more negativity.

Yellow is not a color normally used, or perhaps it is used only in very special circumstances. It is very mentally stimulating and thought to have a temporary brightening effect which, if overdone, can produce exhaustion and subsequent depression.

Atlantean healers normally use only three basic colors—white, blue, and coral. Silver and gold are sometimes used in mental healing (for psychological cases) or for conditions associated with the head and eyes.

Many healers prefer not to visualize any color at all. Although often, as in the case of the cut finger mentioned previously, a clairvoyant will see a color (in this case blue) when the healer has not been consciously visualizing it.

Earlier exercises in color visualization will help to concentrate the mind to a point where these colors can be used. For the purposes of the Atlantean course for "lone healers," it is not necessary. In any case, if one finds it difficult to visualize color, as many people do, just think of the sensation you wish to transmit—hot, cold, soothing, stimulating, cleansing, and so on. Most beginners find it easy to visualize white and blue, and once experienced is gained, colors can either be abandoned or evolved further depending on the direction one's healing abilities take.

CONCLUSION

There are many other color healers and therapists working along these lines, and it is not possible to mention them all. Healing comes in many guises and one has to shop around a bit to find one's own particular wavelength. What may suit one person may suit another, and physical problems of a severe nature may need treatment of an orthodox medical nature. If, however, orthodox treatment can be combined with alternative healing of some kind, it then means that the whole person is being treated on all levels rather than for an isolated and localized medical condition. For those not actually ill, there are still the problems of fatigue, stress, worry, and so on, that prevent one from enjoying life and exploring one's full potential. This is where alternative methods of healing tend to come into their own by providing a wide range of treatments. This is not to discount, of course, the fact that alternative healing methods produce positive cures for all sorts of conditions and often in cases where normal medical treatment has failed. It all depends, as said before, on one finding the right wavelength.

Color is an indispensable factor in our lives. Let us be more aware of it, enjoy it, and exploit it to the fullest—and even if perhaps we can't see some colors all that well, we can still become conscious of their potency in some of the ways outlined in this book. Let's try to make ourselves a more color-full, cheerful, and exciting new world!

ENDNOTES

Chapter 1

1. There is some controversy over the phrase "wine-dark sea." Two Canadian scientists claim that the explanation lies in Greek water, which is strongly alkaline and, when added to wine in certain proportions, tends to turn Greek wine from red to blue. It was commonplace in Homer's day to mix water and wine.
2. Manfred Lurker, *Gods and Symbols of Ancient Egypt* (London: Thames & Hudson, 1980).
3. June Osborne, *Stained Glass in England* (London: Frederick Muller Ltd., 1981).

Chapter 2

1. Faber Birren, *Light, Color and the Environment* (New York: Van Nostrand Reinhold Co. Inc., 1969).
2. Faber Birren, *Color and Human Response* (New York: Van Nostrand Reinhold Co. Inc., 1978).
3. Faber Birrin, *Color: A Survey in Words and Pictures* (New York: University Books, 1963).
4. Theo Gimbel, *Healing Through Colour* (Saffron Walden, U.K.: The C. W. Daniel Co. Ltd., 1980).
5. Birren, *Color and Human Response.*
6. "Science Times," *New York Times,* October 19, 1982.
7. Birren, *Color and Human Response.*

8. Hazel Rossotti, *Colour: Why the World Isn't Grey* (New York: Pelican Books, 1983).
9. "Science Times," *New York Times.*
10. Gimbel, *Healing Through Colour.*
11. Colin Wilson, *Access to Inner Worlds* (London: Rider, 1983).
12. Sheila Ostrander and Lynn Schroeder, *Psychic Discoveries Behind the Iron Curtain* (London: Sphere Books, 1973).
13. Rossotti, *Colour: Why the World Isn't Grey.*

Chapter 3

1. Hazel Rossotti, *Colour: Why the World Isn't Grey* (New York: Pelican Books, 1983).
2. Audrey Kargere, *Color and Personality* (York Beach, Maine: Samuel Weiser Inc., 1979).
3. Faber Birren, *Color and the Human Response* (New York: Van Nostrand Reinhold Co. Inc., 1978).
4. Faber Birren, *Light, Color and the Environment* (New York: Van Nostrand Reinhold Co. Inc., 1969).
5. Max Lüscher, *The Lüscher Colour Test*, trans. by Ian Scott (London: Jonathan Cape Ltd., 1970).

Chapter 4

1. Exodus 34:30.
2. Carlos Castaneda, *A Separate Reality* (New York: Penguin Books, 1973).
3. Thelma Moss, *The Probability of the Impossible* (RKP, 1976).
4. S. G. J. Ouseley, *The Science of the Aura* (London: L. N. Fowler & Co. Ltd., 1949).
5. Jeremy Taylor, *Dream Work* (Romford, U.K.: Fowler Wright Books Ltd., 1983).
6. Charles A. Padgham, *"Colors experienced in dreams."* British Journal of Psychology 66, 1 (1973): 25–28.

Chapter 5

1. F. Ellinger as mentioned in *Color and Human Response,* Faber Birren (New York: Van Nostrand Reinhold Co., Inc., 1978).
2. Annie Wilson and Lilla Bek, *What Color Are You?* (Turnstone Press Ltd., 1982).
3. Mary Anderson, *Colour Healing* (London: The Aquarian Press, 1979).
4. Roland Hunt, *Fragrant and Radiant Healing Symphony* (H. G. White, 1949).

5. Crystal Healing Centre, J. & J. Harvey, Middle Piccadilly, Holwell, Sherborne, Dorset. Tel. Bishops Caundle 468.

6. Francoise Strachan, *Natural Magic* (London: Marshall Cavendish Publications Ltd., 1974).

7. *Healing in the World Today* (Atlanteans Association Ltd., 1977). An Atlantean Study Course including basic instructions on how to heal. Obtainable from the Atlanteans, Runnings Park, Croft Bank, West Malvern, Worcs.

8. Murry Hope, *Practical Techniques of Psychic Self Defense* (London: The Aquarian Press, 1983).

9. *Prediction,* December 1983.

FURTHER
READING

Chapter 1

Bucke R. M., *Cosmic Consciousness*. New York: University Books Inc., 1961.

Cooper, J. C. *An Illustrated Encyclopedia of Traditional Symbols*. London: Thames & Hudson, 1978.

Watson, Lyall. *Lightning Bird*. Dunton Green, U.K.: Coronet Books, 1982.

Wilson, Colin. Access to Inner Worlds. London: Rider, 1983.

Chapter 4

Burr, Harold Saxton. *Blueprint for Immortality*. London: Neville Spearman, 1972.

Castaneda, Carlos. *The Teachings of Don Juan: A Yaqui Way of Knowledge*. New York: Penguin Books, 1974.

Castaneda, Carlos. *Journey to Ixtlan*. New York: Penguin, 1974.

Kilner, Walter J. *The Human Aura*. New York: University Books, 1965.

Long, Max Freedom. *The Secret Science Behind Miracles*. Vista, Calif.: Reasearch Publications, 1948.

Russell, Edward W. *Design for Destiny*. London: Neville Spearman.

Life Outside the Physical Body, Color and Reincarnation. Atlanteans Association Ltd., 1975.

Chapter 5

Gimbel, Theo. *Healing Through Color.* Saffron Walden, U.K.: The C. W. Daniel Co. Ltd., 1980.

Gimbel, Theo. *Key, Lock and Door.* Hygeia Publications, 1976.

Ouseley, S. G. J. *Colour Meditations.* London: L. N. Fowler & Co. Ltd., 1949.

Sturzaker, James. *The Twelve Rays.* London: The Aquarium Press, 1976.

INDEX

Books of Related Interest

Taoist Cosmic Healing
Chi Kung Color Healing Principles for
Detoxification and Rejuvenation
by Mantak Chia

Light: Medicine of the Future
How We Can Use It to Heal Ourselves NOW
by Jacob Liberman, O.D., Ph.D.

Right Brain/Left Brain Reflexology
by Madeleine Turgeon, N.D.

Alchemical Healing
A Guide to Spiritual, Physical, and Transformational Medicine
by Nicki Scully

The Healing Power of Gemstones
In Tantra, Ayurveda, and Astrology
by Harish Johari

The Healing Power of the Mind
Practical Techniques for Health and Empowerment
by Rolf Alexander, M.D.

Healing with Chakra Energy
Restoring the Natural Harmony of the Body
by Lilla Bek & Philippa Pullar

The Book of Ki
A Practical Guide to the Healing Principles of Life Energy
by Mallory Fromm, Ph.D.

INNER TRADITIONS • BEAR & COMPANY
P.O. Box 388
Rochester, VT 05767
1-800-246-8648
www.InnerTraditions.com

Or contact your local bookseller